Primary Care Sports Medicine: Updates and Advances

Guest Editors

JOHN M. MACKNIGHT, MD
DILAAWAR J. MISTRY, MD, ATC

CLINICS IN SPORTS MEDICINE

www.sportsmed.theclinics.com

Consulting Editor
MARK D. MILLER, MD

July 2011 • Volume 30 • Number 3

SAUNDERS an imprint of ELSEVIER, Inc.

W.B. SAUNDERS COMPANY

A Division of Elsevier Inc.

1600 John F. Kennedy Blvd. • Suite 1800 • Philadelphia, Pennsylvania 19103

http://www.theclinics.com

CLINICS IN SPORTS MEDICINE Volume 30, Number 3
July 2011 ISSN 0278-5919, ISBN-13: 978-1-4557-1045-4

Editor: Jessica Demetriou

Clinics in Sports Medicine (ISSN 0278-5919) is published quarterly by Elsevier Inc., 360 Park Avenue South, New York, NY 10010-1710. Months of issue are January, April, July, and October. Business and Editorial Offices: 1600 John F. Kennedy Blvd., Ste. 1800, Philadelphia, PA 19103-2899. Customer Service Office: 3251 Riverport Lane, Maryland Heights, MO 63043. Periodicals postage paid at New York, NY and additional mailing offices. Subscription prices are $297.00 per year (US individuals), $466.00 per year (US institutions), $147.00 per year (US students), $337.00 per year (Canadian individuals), $563.00 per year (Canadian institutions), $205.00 (Canadian students), $409.00 per year (foreign individuals), $563.00 per year (foreign institutions), and $205.00 per year (foreign students). Foreign air speed delivery is included in all *Clinics* subscription prices. All prices are subject to change without notice. **POSTMASTER:** Send address changes to *Clinics in Sports Medicine*, Elsevier Health Sciences Division, Subscription Customer Service, 3251 Riverport Lane, Maryland Heights, MO 63043. Customer Service (orders, claims, online, change of address): Elsevier Health Sciences Division, Subscription Customer Service, 3251 Riverport Lane, Maryland Heights, MO 63043. Tel: 1-800-654-2452 (U.S. and Canada); 314-447-8871 (outside U.S. and Canada). Fax: 314-447-8029. E-mail: journalscustomerservice-usa@elsevier.com (for print support); journalsonlinesupport-usa@elsevier.com (for online support).

Reprints. For copies of 100 or more of articles in this publication, please contact the Commercial Reprints Department, Elsevier Inc., 360 Park Avenue South, New York, NY 10010-1710. Tel.: 212-633-3812; Fax: 212-462-1935; E-mail: reprints@elsevier.com.

Clinics in Sports Medicine is covered in *MEDLINE/PubMed (Index Medicus) Current Contents/Clinical Medicine, Excerpta Medica,* and *ISI/Biomed.*

Printed and bound by CPI Group (UK) Ltd, Croydon, CR0 4YY

Transferred to Digital Print 2011

Contributors

CONSULTING EDITOR

MARK D. MILLER, MD
S. Ward Casscells Professor of Orthopaedic Surgery, University of Virginia, Charlottesville, Virginia; Team Physician, James Madison University, Harrisonburg, Virginia

GUEST EDITORS

JOHN M. MACKNIGHT, MD
Associate Professor, Clinical Internal Medicine and Orthopaedic Surgery, University of Virginia Health System; Primary Care Team Physician and Co-Medical Director, University of Virginia Sports Medicine, Charlottesville, Virginia

DILAAWAR J. MISTRY, MD, ATC
Associate Professor, Physical Medicine and Rehabilitation and Internal Medicine, University of Virginia Health System; Team Physician and Co-Medical Director, University of Virginia Sports Medicine, Charlottesville, Virginia; Team Physician, U.S.A. Swimming, Colorado Springs, Colorado

AUTHORS

ROBERT W. BATTLE, MD, FACC
Associate Professor of Medicine and Pediatrics, Co-Director, Adult Congenital Heart Clinic; Head Team Cardiologist, University of Virginia Athletic Programs; Division of Cardiology, University of Virginia Health System, Charlottesville, Virginia

LESLIE J. BONCI, MPH, RD, CSSD, LDN
Director, Sports Medicine Nutrition, Department of Orthopedic Surgery and the Center for Sports Medicine, University of Pittsburgh, Pittsburgh, Pennsylvania

DONNA K. BROSHEK, PhD
Associate Professor of Psychiatry and Neurobehavioral Sciences, Neurocognitive Assessment Laboratory, Department of Psychiatry and Neurobehavioral Sciences, University of Virginia School of Medicine, Charlottesville, Virginia

MARIO CIOCCA, MD
Director of Sports Medicine and Assistant Professor of Internal Medicine and Orthopaedics, James A Taylor Campus Health Service, UNC Sports Medicine, University of North Carolina, Chapel Hill, North Carolina

BRIAN DONOHUE, DO
Sports Medicine Fellow, Sports Medicine Fellowship, Resurrection Medical Center, Chicago, Illinois

E. RANDY EICHNER, MD
Former Team Internist, OU Sooner Football; Professor Emeritus of Medicine, University of Oklahoma Health Sciences Center, Oklahoma City, Oklahoma

ALI ESFANDIARI, PhD
Postdoctoral Fellow, Neurocognitive Assessment Laboratory, Department of Psychiatry and Neurobehavioral Sciences, University of Virginia School of Medicine, Charlottesville, Virginia

JASON R. FREEMAN, PhD
Associate Professor of Psychiatry and Neurobehavioral Sciences, Neurocognitive Assessment Laboratory, Department of Psychiatry and Neurobehavioral Sciences, University of Virginia School of Medicine, Charlottesville, Virginia

DANIEL HERMAN, MD, PhD
Resident, Department of Physical Medicine and Rehabilitation, University of Virginia Health System, Charlottesville, Virginia

ANNE Z. HOCH, DO
Department of Physical Medicine and Rehabilitation; Professor and Director, Women's Sports Medicine Program, Department of Orthopaedic Surgery, Sports Medicine Center, Medical College of Wisconsin, Milwaukee, Wisconsin

CARRIE A. JAWORSKI, MD
Director of Intercollegiate Sports Medicine and Head Team Physician, Intercollegiate Sports Medicine, Northwestern University, Evanston; Assistant Professor of Family and Community Medicine, Feinberg School of Medicine, Northwestern University, Chicago, Illinois

JOSHUA KLUETZ, DO
Sports Medicine Fellow, Sports Medicine Fellowship, Resurrection Medical Center, Chicago, Illinois

RONNIE LANEY, MD
Department of Family Medicine, University of North Carolina, Chapel Hill, North Carolina

ARIANE L. SMITH MACHIN, PhD
Licensed Clinical and Sport Psychologist, Women's Sports Medicine Program, Sports Medicine Center, Medical College of Wisconsin, Milwaukee, Wisconsin

JOHN M. MACKNIGHT, MD
Associate Professor, Clinical Internal Medicine and Orthopaedic Surgery, University of Virginia Health System; Primary Care Team Physician and Co-Medical Director, University of Virginia Sports Medicine, Charlottesville, Virginia

SRIJOY MAHAPATRA, BSEE, MD, FHRS
Assistant Professor of Medicine and Biomedical Engineering, Cardiovascular Research Director, University of Virginia Athletic Programs; Division of Cardiology, University of Virginia Health System, Charlottesville, Virginia

ROHIT MALHOTRA, MD
Division of Cardiology; Electrophysiology Fellowship Program, University of Virginia Health System, Charlottesville, Virginia

DILAAWAR J. MISTRY, MD, ATC
Associate Professor, Physical Medicine and Rehabilitation and Internal Medicine, University of Virginia Health System; Team Physician and Co-Medical Director, University of Virginia Sports Medicine, Charlottesville, Virginia; Team Physician, U.S.A. Swimming, Colorado Springs, Colorado

JESSE W. PARR, MD
Assistant Clinical Professor, Department of Pediatrics, Texas A&M Health Science Center; Team Physician, Texas A&M University, College Station, Texas

ETHAN N. SALIBA, PhD, PT, ATC
Adjunct Assistant Professor of Physical Medicine and Rehabilitation and Orthopedic Surgery, University of Virginia Health System; Department of Athletics, University of Virginia, Charlottesville, Virginia

CRAIG K. SETO, MD, FAAFP, CAQ-SM
Associate Professor of Family Medicine and Primary Care Sports Medicine Fellowship Director, Department of Family Medicine, University of Virginia Health System, Charlottesville, Virginia

HARRY STAFFORD, MD
Assistant Professor, Family Medicine and Orthopaedics, Team Physician, James A Taylor Campus Health Service, UNC Sports Medicine, University of North Carolina, Chapel Hill, North Carolina

AMY E. STROMWALL, MD
Summit Orthopedics Ltd, St Paul, Minnesota; Team Physician, U.S.A. Swimming, Colorado Springs, Colorado

JONATHON D. TRUWIT, MD, MBA
E. Cato Drash Professor of Medicine; Senior Associate Dean for Clinical Affairs; Chief Medical Officer; Division of Pulmonary and Critical Care Medicine, University of Virginia Health System, Charlottesville, Virginia

MAX M. WEDER, MD
Assistant Professor of Medicine, Division of Pulmonary and Critical Care Medicine, University of Virginia Health System, Charlottesville, Virginia

KARIE N. ZACH, MD
Fellow, Department of Orthopaedic Surgery, Sports Medicine Center; Department of Physical Medicine and Rehabilitation, Medical College of Wisconsin, Milwaukee, Wisconsin

Contents

> The evolution of the preparticipation physical examination (PPE) in the United States continues to advance. In May 2010, the fourth edition of the *Preparticipation Physical Examination Evaluation* (PPE-4) monograph was published. The monograph is a product reflecting the collaborative efforts of 6 author societies. This article provides a brief historical review of the PPE and then highlights the recent changes and updates contained in the PPE-4 monograph, including cardiovascular screening in athletes. New recommendations to include the PPE in all well-child care visits and the need to develop a nationwide standard for the PPE are discussed.

> This article addresses programmatic cardiovascular screening and evaluation of the elite athlete at the intercollegiate, national team, professional, and Olympic levels. Although much of this content may apply to high-school and recreational sports at large, it is not specifically designed to address athletes participating in all sports activities.

> Exercise is rarely limited by pulmonary causes in normal individuals. Cardiac output and peripheral muscle disease are usually the limiting factors. Although minute ventilation rises steeply during exercise, normal individuals maintain a substantial breathing reserve. Exercise in patients, however, can be limited by pulmonary disorders. Acute pulmonary causes (exercise-induced bronchospasm, vocal cord dysfunction, exercise-induced anaphylaxis, and exercise-induced urticaria) or chronic disorders (obstructive and restrictive lung disorders) reduce exercise tolerance. Exercise testing has proved the mainstay for diagnosis and treatment of these disorders.

> This article highlights the exertional-sickling collapse syndrome in athletes with sickle cell trait (SCT). It covers all aspects of this syndrome, including

pathophysiology, new research on microcirculatory changes, clinical features, differential diagnosis, prevention, and treatment. Also covered in this article are other clinical concerns for athletes with SCT, including lumbar myonecrosis, splenic infarction, hematuria, hyposthenuria, and venous thromboembolism. The final section offers practical points on athletes with sickling hemoglobinopathies more serious than SCT.

Although there are numerous benefits to women from athletic participation, a complex combination of endocrine and metabolic factors exaggerates risk for a serious health concern: the female athlete triad. The purpose of this article is to provide updates on new issues related to the triad, specifically the relationship between athletic-associated amenorrhea and endothelial dysfunction—a potential fourth component to the triad that is a concern for future cardiovascular risk, public health issues, and athletic performance. Folic acid should be considered a potential safe and inexpensive therapeutic treatment to restore endothelial-dependent vasodilation.

Athletes are susceptible to the same infections as the general population. However, special considerations often need to be taken into account when dealing with an athlete who has contracted an infectious disease. Health care providers need to consider how even common illnesses can affect an athlete's performance, the communicability of the illness to team members, and precautions/contraindications related to athletic participation. Recent advances in the prevention, diagnosis, and/or management of frequently encountered illnesses, as well as certain conditions that warrant special attention in the athletic setting, are discussed in detail.

Attention-deficit/hyperactivity disorder (ADHD) is a brain-based behavioral disorder with heterogeneous expression affecting quality of life. Some affected individuals may not experience obvious impairment until after arrival at college. The incidence of ADHD may be increased among athletes who participate at the elite level. Neurotransmitters involved in ADHD also are involved in central fatigue, and fatigue research using medications used to treat ADHD suggests that endurance performance and thermoregulation are affected in ways that may put athletes taking these medications at risk. More information is needed on the effect on exercise of long-term administration of ADHD medication.

This article reviews psychiatric/psychological issues in the athletic training room, including recognition of these issues and a framework for management. Because the majority of research has been conducted in college settings, most of the issues discussed are presented in the context of college sports, although the results generalize to other athletic arenas. Greater awareness of psychological issues, empirical research, and education about mental health issues in the sports medicine community are clearly needed.

Athletes use a variety of substances for the treatment of pain, injury, common illnesses, or to gain an advantage in competition. A growing concern is that many young athletes may use potentially dangerous, but legal, medications without consulting health professionals. Physicians providing care for athletes should be aware of any medications that an athlete is taking and how these substances may interact with performance, exercise, environment, and other medicines. Moreover, it is vital that physicians are familiar with these medications so that athletes are properly educated on the potential benefits and/or risks, and how each substance may affect the body.

To perform at the highest level of international competition, athletes need to maximize rest during long travel, and expeditiously overcome the detrimental effects of "jet lag" (JL). The negative effects of JL may be alleviated by adopting a multimodality approach, including the judicious use of melatonin and other pharmacologic agents to aid re-entrainment and improve sleep characteristics. Strict compliance with anti-doping policy is pivotal before and during competition. There have been several recent updates regarding the use of selected medications, which mandate constant vigilance by sports medicine personnel to both evaluate drug efficacy and judiciously prescribe approved medications. It is critical that medical staff maintain familiarity and awareness on a continual basis to effectively educate athletes and support staff.

Despite many advances in nutritional knowledge and dietary practices, sports nutrition-associated issues, such as fatigue, loss of strength and stamina, loss of speed, and problems with weight management and inadequate energy intake, are common. Sound nutritional practices and well-designed patterns of eating are not awarded the same priority as training and many athletes fail to recognize that poor eating habits or suboptimal hydration choices may detract from athletic performance. Those who care for athletes and active individuals must take an active role in their nutritional well-being. This article reviews the present generally accepted principles for nutritional management in sport.

RELATED INTEREST

Clinics in Podiatric Medicine and Surgery, January 2011 (Volume 28, Issue 1)
Foot and Ankle Athletic Injuries
Bob Baravarian, DPM, FACFAS, *Guest Editor*
Available at: http://www.podiatric.theclinics.com/

VISIT THE CLINICS ONLINE!

Access your subscription at:
www.theclinics.com

Foreword

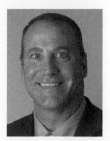

Mark D. Miller, MD
Consulting Editor

Early in my tenure as consulting editor for *Clinics in Sports Medicine*, I received some criticism for focusing too much on orthopedic-related issues at the exclusion of medical-related issues. I "get it" now and have tried to provide a good balance of subjects for *Clinics*. I realized that we haven't had an update on some critical medical issues that are evolving, so I asked my "go to" colleagues, who have done an excellent job as guest editors in the past, to put together this issue. As always, they have come through with flying colors! The issue, much like the team doctor's first duty, begins with the preparticipation physical exam. Drs MacKnight and Mistry then have put together key updates on a variety of medical issues from cardiopulmonary, to infectious disease, to psychological and nutritional issues, and even an update on the international athlete. They are to be congratulated for pulling together such a diverse and informative issue that should be of tremendous benefit to all medical providers who care for athletes. The timing of this issue is perfect... just in time to launch into a new college season! Go [insert team of your choice here]!

Mark D. Miller, MD
S. Ward Casscells Professor of Orthopaedic Surgery
University of Virginia
Team Physician, James Madison University
400 Ray C. Hunt Drive, Suite 330
Charlottesville, VA 22908-0159, USA

E-mail address:
mdm3p@virginia.edu

Clin Sports Med 30 (2011) xi
doi:10.1016/j.csm.2011.05.002
0278-5919/11/$ – see front matter © 2011 Elsevier Inc. All rights reserved.

sportsmed.theclinics.com

Preface

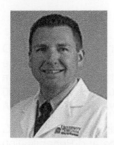 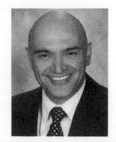

John M. MacKnight, MD   Dilaawar J. Mistry, MD, ATC
Guest Editors

No area of medicine is static, and sports medicine is no exception. In recent years, the management of medical conditions, including the use of medications, therapies, and diagnostic modalities, has been debated and emerged, advanced, and changed significantly. Thus, when we first contemplated putting together this most recent issue in the *Clinics in Sports Medicine* series, we asked ourselves, "What would be most valuable to the busy sports medicine care provider?" "How is the busy practitioner to keep up with dynamic change?" Almost instantly, the answer that made the most sense to both of us was to produce an issue that encompasses the areas of greatest interest, recent changes, and notable developments.

In this issue we have assembled a distinguished group of contributing authors with expertise in a broad array of sports medicine topics. You will find updated information about the preparticipation physical exam process, recent changes associated with the release of the PPE-4, and future directions that may be pursued in this crucial step in safeguarding the health and well-being of athletic individuals. Along those same lines, we present new information regarding a number of critical cardiovascular issues in athletes. As the use of psycho-stimulant drugs for attention deficit disorder (ADD) has reached epidemic proportions, we felt it vital to present a comprehensive article on ADD and the management challenges faced in the athletic population. You will find up-to-date information in the areas of sports nutrition and mental health concerns in athletes as well. Each of these areas has become a more prominent concern in training rooms and clinics at all sports levels. Rounding out this issue are articles addressing pulmonary issues in athletes, unique considerations in the international and traveling athlete, a review of sickle cell trait, female athlete triad and eating disorders, infectious diseases, and the athlete's pharmacy. We have tried hard to encompass the commonly encountered issues in an athletic training room setting, with a focus on those areas that have undergone rapid or significant change in recent years.

We hope that this *Clinics* issue, which is dedicated to "Updates and Advances in Sports Medicine," will be a valuable addition to your sports medicine library and help you stay abreast of the current literature in our rapidly emerging world of sports medicine. If it is true to its intent, it will assist you in feeling up to date with respect to the present standard of care in many crucial areas in sports medicine, while also laying a foundation for future areas of growth and change. Similarly, we hope that

Clin Sports Med 30 (2011) xiii–xiv
doi:10.1016/j.csm.2011.05.001
0278-5919/11/$ – see front matter © 2011 Elsevier Inc. All rights reserved.
sportsmed.theclinics.com

you will enjoy this work as much as we have enjoyed assembling it. May your care of athletes prosper and may you find joy, as we do, in playing a vital role in the health, well-being, and success of athletes and active individuals.

Cheers!

John M. MacKnight, MD
Department of Medicine
University of Virginia Health System
415 Ray C. Hunt Drive, Suite 2100
Charlottesville, VA 22908-0671, USA

Dilaawar J. Mistry, MD, ATC
Departments of Athletics and Physical Medicine and Rehabilitation
University of Virginia Health System
545 Ray C. Hunt Drive, Suite 240, PO Box 801004
Charlottesville, VA 22908-1004, USA

E-mail addresses:
JM9M@hscmail.mcc.virginia.edu (J.M. MacKnight)
DM5F@hscmail.mcc.virginia.edu (D.J. Mistry)

The Preparticipation Physical Examination: An Update

Craig K. Seto, MD, CAQ-SM

KEYWORDS

• Preparticipation physical examination • Evaluation
• Sports medicine • Athletes

The evolution of the preparticipation physical examination (PPE) in the United States continues to advance. In May 2010, the fourth edition of the *Preparticipation Physical Evaluation* (PPE-4) monograph was published. The monograph is a product reflecting the collaborative efforts of 6 author societies: American Academy of Family Physicians, American Academy of Pediatrics, American College of Sports Medicine, American Medical Society for Sports Medicine, American Orthopaedic Society for Sports Medicine, and American Osteopathic Academy of Sports Medicine. The content and recommendations within the monograph are based on a comprehensive review of current literature, position and consensus statements, policies, and expert opinion, along with an extensive peer review process. As such, the PPE-4 monograph can be viewed as the current standard in regards to the performance of the PPE in the United States.[1] This article provides a brief historical review of the PPE and then highlights the recent changes and updates contained in the PPE-4 monograph, including cardiovascular screening in athletes. New recommendations to include the PPE in all well-child care visits and the need to develop a nationwide standard for the PPE are discussed.

HISTORICAL REVIEW OF THE PPE

For many years physicians have been conducting PPEs on athletes before competition. The first generation of PPE began approximately 40 years ago and consisted of a simple process termed the "triple H." The evaluation consisted of 3 components: (1) how are you, (2) heart auscultation, and (3) hernia check. The obvious goal of the examination was to detect heart murmurs and asymptomatic hernias. The second generation of the PPE advanced slightly by including questions regarding the past medical history and a urinalysis. A limited physical examination was performed and a clearance form was provided to be signed by the physician. The third generation

---

Department of Family Medicine, University of Virginia Health System, PO Box 800729, Charlottesville, VA 22908, USA
E-mail address: cks2n@virginia.edu

Clin Sports Med 30 (2011) 491–501
doi:10.1016/j.csm.2011.03.008
0278-5919/11/$ – see front matter © 2011 Elsevier Inc. All rights reserved.

of the PPE brought about the most significant advancement in the PPE process. It began in 1992 when the first PPE monograph was published through the collaborative efforts of 5 medical societies: American Academy of Family Physicians, American Academy of Pediatrics, American Medical Society of Sports Medicine, American Orthopaedic Society for Sports Medicine, and American Osteopathic Academy of Sports Medicine. The monograph provided a comprehensive guide for the set up and performance of the PPE. It defined the goals and objectives for the PPE along with recommendations for the setting, timing, and structure of the PPE process. The monograph included a history form to be completed by the athlete and a physical examination form with recommendations for clearance. The authors of the monograph hoped to set a standard for the performance of the PPE that would be adopted nationwide. Unfortunately, despite the intentions of the authors, a nationwide standard has never been established.[2–4]

In 1996 the American Heart Association (AHA) consensus panel published its recommendations for performing cardiovascular screening in young athletes. These recommendations were updated by the AHA in 2007 and are the current standard for cardiovascular screening of young athletes in the United States.[5,6] The authors of the PPE monograph have endorsed the AHA recommendations since their initial publication in 1996. The 2007 AHA recommendations for cardiovascular screening have been incorporated into the current PPE-4 monograph. The monograph represents the standard for the performance of the PPE in young athletes. It is a practical and effective screening tool for physicians that can stand alone as a screening examination or can be incorporated into a routine preventive visit.[1,2]

GOALS OF THE PPE

Since the initial publication of the *Preparticipation Physical Evaluation* monograph in 1992, the main goal has been to promote the health and safety of athletes in training and competition and not to exclude them from competition. This goal remains the same today and is ultimately facilitated through the primary and secondary objectives.

1. The primary objectives of the PPE
    To detect potentially life-threatening or disabling medical or musculoskeletal conditions
    To screen for medical or musculoskeletal conditions that may predispose an athlete to injury or illness during training or competition.
2. The secondary objectives of the PPE
    To determine general health
    To serve as an entry point into the health care system for adolescents
    To provide an opportunity to initiate discussion on health-related topics.[1]

Controversy on the Effectiveness of PPE

Traditionally, the PPE has been used as a screening tool to identify injuries, illness, or factors that might place the athlete or others at risk for illness or injury. However, there is significant controversy regarding the effectiveness of the PPE as a screening tool. For a screening tool to be effective it must be able to identify diseases or processes in athletes at a point when the medical issue can be positively impacted upon. Additionally, it must be sensitive, practical, and affordable. Current research fails to demonstrate that the PPE has had any effect on the morbidity or mortality of athletes overall. Data to support its effectiveness as a screening tool is also lacking. Despite the controversy and lack of evidence of its efficacy, PPEs are widely performed throughout the United States, with nearly every state requiring some form of PPE for scholastic athletes. The National Federation of State High School Associations considers the PPE a prerequisite to sports participation. At the collegiate level, the National Collegiate Athletic Association (NCAA) recommends, and most institutions require, a PPE before entrance to the program. Also, programs like Special Olympics require a PPE for its athletes before competing.[1]

The author societies acknowledge the concerns surrounding the PPE but still contend that when the PPE is thoroughly and consistently performed and supervised by qualified and licensed physicians, it may be an effective tool in identifying medical and orthopedic conditions that might affect an athlete's ability to participate safely in sport. Additionally, the PPE can also serve as an important component of adolescent health care. In many adolescent athletes, the PPE may serve as their only contact with a medical provider in a given year. The PPE could therefore serve as an opportunity to facilitate general health care, update immunizations, and establish a medical home.[1]

A Need for Standardization of the PPE

In the United States, there continues to be no national standard for the performance of the preparticipation physical examination despite a recommendation supporting this from all previous monograph authors. Currently, the requirements regarding the length, comprehensiveness, and content of the PPE is determined by each state. The state also determines the type of provider who is licensed to perform the PPE. As a result, the PPE process varies significantly from state to state in regards to scope, content, and training or expertise of provider performing the examination.[1] Several studies have documented significant inconsistency in the content of state PPE forms used at the high school level. A survey study of state high school PPE forms in 1998 found that 40% provided inadequate cardiovascular screening based on the 1996 AHA recommendations. Additionally, only 17% of states had forms that included all components of the AHA recommendations. Eight states did not offer an approved PPE form to guide physicians, and one state had no requirement at all for a PPE. A follow-up study in 2005 revealed a significant improvement with 81% of states having an adequate PPE form. The most recent study in 2009 found that 85% of states had PPE forms that reflected the outdated 1996 AHA guidelines for cardiovascular screening.[7,8]

The variation in the PPE process from state to state has been a significant barrier to determining the effectiveness of the PPE in the United States. The authors of the 2010 monograph have strongly recommended that the United States adopt a standardized approach to the performance of the PPE. A nationwide standard would allow for meaningful data collection and provide an evidence base to assist in evaluating the efficacy of the PPE process. Changes made in the PPE could then be based on evidence and outcome data.[9] This process is the best way to truly determine the effectiveness of our current system and make meaningful changes to improve it.

The PPE-4 monograph could serve as the standard to be adopted and implemented in each state nationwide. The author societies have made the history, physical examination, and clearance forms freely available for download on the Internet at www.ppesportsevaluation.org/evalform.pdf. Unfortunately, the National Federation of State High School Associations lacks the authority to mandate standardization of the PPE across its member states. Therefore, each state would need to adopt and use the PPE-4 as its own before standardization could occur in the United States. The recently formed Campaign and Coalition for Youth Sports Health and Safety has joined in the efforts for standardization. They have strongly urged the sports and medical communities to adopt the guidelines in the PPE-4 monograph and bring about a uniform process for the PPE in the United States.[10]

REVIEWING THE PPE-4 MONOGRAPH
Overview

In the fourth edition of the PPE monograph, the authors have reviewed and updated recommendations on important issues, such as cardiovascular screening and concussion in sport. The monograph has been significantly expanded and provides in-depth reviews of the relevant medical conditions and issues pertaining to athletic sports participation. Sections have been organized according to system and include the history questions that pertain to them, with an explanation of the importance and rationale underlying each question. The monograph has added a comprehensive section on the female athlete to highlight their unique considerations. Physicians will find the monograph to be an invaluable resource and effective clinical tool to assist and guide in the performance of the PPE.[1]

Re-emphasizing the Importance of the History Questions

The medical history is the most sensitive and specific component of the PPE for detecting conditions that affect participation in sports. More than 75% of the important medical and orthopedic conditions affecting athletes can be identified by asking the right historical questions. The monograph authors view the history questions as the most important component of the PPE. As such, they have rewritten and expanded the questionnaire that now includes more than 50 questions. The authors have organized the questionnaire by system making it more user friendly. It is recommended that parents assist in the completion of the questionnaire to help ensure accuracy. The authors have included a supplemental education section to help parents and athletes better understand the significance of the questions and underscore the importance of answering them honestly.[1]

NEW RECOMMENDATIONS IN THE PPE-4
Promoting Health and Fitness for all Children

The authors have made a bold new recommendation to make the PPE part of every routine well-child and adolescent care visit. The authors explain that physicians should be recommending exercise and activity to every child, not just those participating in organized sports. If physicians are going to recommend and promote exercise to all children, then those children should be offered a PPE to help ensure their health and safety during exercise and activity. Currently, most children do not undergo a formal PPE until they reach middle school when it is required for participation in sports. However, before middle school, children involved in athletics or sports do so with little or no formal PPE before participation. Likewise, many children and adolescents participate in vigorous exercise and activities regularly on the playground and in physical education classes. These children are at no less risk of illness or injury while exercising, but most are not offered a formal PPE. This obvious disparity has gone unnoticed for years, but now has been recognized[11] and is the basis for the new recommendation. With childhood obesity reaching epidemic level, promoting health and fitness for all children should be the goal and consistent message from all physicians.[1]

Promoting a Medical Home for all Athletes

The PPE writing group feels that the PPE should ideally be performed in the office of the athlete's primary care physician who is familiar with them and their medical history. The continuity of care and familiarity, combined with a complete medical record, will decrease the likelihood of missing significant medical conditions or concerning family history. The setting also offers privacy and the opportunity to discuss more sensitive issues, including alcohol, tobacco, and drug use and feelings of stress or depression. Risk-taking behaviors related to the use of seatbelts, helmets, and safe sexual practices are more likely to cause harm in the adolescent than sports participation.[1,5] These questions are included on the physical examination form to serve as prompts for further conversation. The authors realize that many young athletes do not have a personal physician, and for many, the PPE is their only contact with a medical provider during the year. This limited exposure to the health care system is another reason to recommend that the PPE be performed in the office of a physician who can provide a medical home for the athlete. If the PPE process must be performed outside the office setting, as a coordinated medical team, it is recommended that physicians perform a complete PPE on an athlete as a one-on-one encounter rather than splitting the examination into different stations based on body system. Mass PPE screenings set up in high school gymnasiums that offer little or no privacy are highly discouraged.[1]

ADDRESSING CONTROVERSY
Cardiovascular Screening in Athletes

The authors of the PPE-4 acknowledge the current ongoing controversy regarding the most effective way to screen young athletes for underlying cardiovascular abnormalities. The monograph provides a comprehensive overview of sudden cardiac death (SCD) in young athletes and the current controversy regarding cardiovascular screening. The authors provide a thorough and balanced review of this important issue including the arguments for and against the routine use of noninvasive tests, such as the electrocardiogram (ECG) and echocardiogram in the PPE.

Controversy Surrounding Cardiovascular Screening

The current controversy in the United States surrounds the benefit of using noninvasive screening tests, such as the ECG, in the routine screening of athletes. The current cardiovascular screening recommendations in the United States call for a detailed personal and family history and focused physical examination, but do not recommend the routine use of ECG. However, recently, the European Society of Cardiology and the International Olympic Committee have both endorsed the routine use of the ECG in addition to a detailed medical history and physical examination in the preparticipation screening of athletes. These recommendations are based on the published success of the Italian national preparticipation screening system that uses the ECG in addition to a detailed medical history and physical examination for routine screening of all athletes. In Italy, all preparticipation examinations take place in designated screening centers and are performed by specifically trained sports physicians with expertise in cardiovascular screening and ECG interpretation. Using this system, Italian authors have reported an 89% reduction in the incidence of SCD in screened athletes over a 25-year period. Corrado and colleagues[12] published these results in 2006. The Italian authors credit the ECG and its superior ability to identify athletes with underlying cardiovascular abnormalities as the main reason for the success of the system. Since the publication of these studies, many have argued for the adoption of such a system in the United States.[13–15]

AHA Recommendations Regarding Use of ECG

In 2007, the AHA consensus panel convened and after a careful review of the available studies in the literature recommended against the use of the ECG in the routine screening of athletes. The AHA felt the addition of the ECG was not a feasible option for mass universal screening in the United States because of the low prevalence of disease, poor sensitivity, high false positive rates, poor cost-effectiveness, and lack of properly trained clinicians to interpret the results.[6] Despite the AHA recommendations, this topic continues to be the focus of intense study and debate. This area is rapidly evolving and will require physicians to stay abreast of the latest recommendations as new information becomes available.[1]

PPE-4 RECOMMENDATIONS FOR CARDIOVASCULAR SCREENING IN ATHLETES

The PPE-4 monograph follows the AHA 2007 consensus guidelines that recommend

1. A complete and targeted personal and family history
2. A physical examination designed to identify or raise suspicion for cardiovascular diseases known to cause SCD
3. ECG and echocardiogram are NOT recommended for the routine screening of asymptomatic athletes.

PPE cardiovascular screening questions were developed to elicit responses that may indicate the presence of a serious cardiac condition and lead to further investigation. Parent or guardian verification is recommended for high school and middle school athletes to ensure accuracy. Use of a standardized and detailed questionnaire is strongly recommended to assist health care providers in performing a comprehensive cardiovascular risk assessment.

Identifying Channelopathies

The authors have added additional cardiovascular questions to the questionnaire in an attempt to identify individuals with rare electrical cardiac abnormalities termed *channelopathies*. This group of cardiac disorders accounts for approximately 3% of SCD in athletes, but could account for many cases of sudden unexplained death in athletes.

The channelopathies include

1. Long QT syndrome, catecholaminergic polymorphic ventricular tachycardia
2. Wolff-Parkinson-White syndrome and Brugada syndrome.

Individuals with underlying channelopathies will frequently have

1. A *personal history* of syncope, seizures, or arrhythmias
2. A *family history* of unexpected or unexplained sudden death, drowning or near drowning, unexplained motor vehicle accident, unexplained seizures, or sudden infant death.

PPE PERSONAL HISTORY QUESTIONS

1. Have you ever passed out or nearly passed out during or after exercise?
2. Have you ever had discomfort, pain, tightness, or pressure in your chest during exercise?
3. Does your heart ever race or skip beats (irregular beats) during exercise?
4. Has a doctor every told you that you have any heart problems (high blood pressure, high cholesterol, a heart murmur, a heart infection, Kawasaki disease, or other)?
5. Has a doctor ever ordered a test for your heart (for example, ECG or echocardiogram)?
6. Do you get lightheaded or feel more short of breath than expected during exercise?

7. Have you ever had an unexplained seizure?
8. Do you get more tired or short of breath more quickly than your friends during exercise?

PPE FAMILY HISTORY QUESTIONS

1. Has any family member or relative died of heart problems or had any unexpected or unexplained sudden death before 50 years of age, including drowning, unexplained car accident, or sudden infant death syndrome?
2. Does anyone in your family have hypertrophic cardiomyopathy, Marfan syndrome, arrhythmogenic right ventricular cardiomyopathy, long QT syndrome, short QT syndrome, Brugada syndrome, or catecholaminergic polymorphic ventricular tachycardia?
3. Does anyone in your family have a heart problem, pacemaker, or implanted defibrillator?
4. Has anyone in your family had unexplained fainting, unexplained seizures, or near drowning?

THE CARDIOVASCULAR PHYSICAL EXAMINATION

1. Dynamic auscultation for heart murmurs
   Should be performed in both the supine and standing position or with Valsalva maneuver (The standing position is preferred to help accentuate the murmur of hypertrophic cardiomyopathy.)
2. Palpation of radial and femoral pulses to exclude aortic coarctation
3. Examination for physical stigmata of Marfan syndrome
   Kyphoscoliosis, high arched palate, pectus excavatum, arachnodactyly
   Arm span greater than height, hyperlaxity, myopia, mitral valve prolapse, and aortic insufficiency
4. Brachial artery blood pressure taken in the sitting position.

Recommendations for Further Investigation

Any athlete with symptoms of exertional syncope, near syncope, chest pain, palpitations, or excessive exertional dyspnea will require a thorough cardiovascular evaluation to exclude underlying heart disease. They should be restricted from any athletic participation until this workup is completed.[1]

Limitations of PPE Cardiovascular Evaluation

The authors remind clinicians that currently there are no outcomes-based studies that demonstrate the effectiveness of the current PPE in preventing or detecting athletes at risk for sudden death.[1]

IMPORTANT MEDICAL ISSUES AFFECTING ATHLETIC PARTICIPATION
Concussion in Athletes

The monograph provides an updated review of this topic to help providers better understand the most important issues related to concussions in sport. The review includes common signs and symptoms, diagnosis, management, and the recommendation for a graded return-to-play protocol. Important sequelae associated with concussions, including second impact syndrome, postconcussive syndrome, and long-term neurologic dysfunction, are also covered. The monograph also includes a copy of the Sport Concussion Assessment Tool 2 in the appendix to assist with the evaluation of athletes with suspected concussion. Each section provides a key summary of bulleted points highlighting the most important aspects of this condition.

Important key points related to concussion

1. Concussions are common, underreported, and many times not recognized.
2. Loss of consciousness is not required for a concussion to occur.
3. No athlete who sustains a concussion should return to play until completely asymptomatic.
4. Once an athlete is asymptomatic, they should undergo a graded return-to-play protocol (included in the monograph).
5. Athletes younger than 18 years take longer to recover than older athletes.
6. Computerized neuropsychological testing is most effective when a baseline test has been performed for comparison.
7. Decisions to return to play following a concussion must be individualized.[1]

Sickle Cell Trait in Athletes

There is currently no recommendation for universal screening in athletes; however, the NCAA recently instituted screening for athletes if their sickle cell trait status is not already known. Clinicians should be aware of the main concerns related to this condition.

Important key points related to sickle cell trait

1. Sickle cell trait occurs in approximately 8% of black Americans and 0.01% to 0.05% of Caucasians. It is non-life threatening in normal circumstances; however, during strenuous activity, especially in hot humid environments or at altitude, there have been case reports of sudden death in athletes with sickle cell trait.
2. The US military has reported a 20-fold increase in risk of sudden death in recruits with sickle cell trait. Death results from the complications of sickling, including rhabdomyolysis, profound acidosis, acute renal failure, and multi-organ system failure.
3. Athletes with sickle cell trait should maintain adequate hydration and be advised to avoid strenuous exercise that leads to muscle pain during early season sprints.[1]

The Female Athlete

This new section of the monograph provides an excellent review of the unique issues in female athletes that affect their health and participation. The PPE questions target these issues. A discussion regarding clearance recommendations for athletes with disordered eating and the female athletic triad are included.

Important key points related to the female athlete

1. Disordered eating is common in female athletes.
2. Eating disorders and energy imbalance may be associated with amenorrhea, persistent injury, recurrent injury, or stress fractures.
3. Female athletes with menstrual dysfunction have longer interruptions of training than those with regular cycles.
4. Vitamin D deficiency is becoming increasingly common in female athletes because of inadequate dietary intake or reduced exposure to sunlight.

5. *Musculoskeletal problems*: Female athletes are at higher risk for noncontact anterior cruciate ligament injury, recurrent patellar dislocation, patellofemoral disorder, and stress fractures.
6. *Neurologic*: Female athletes have higher rates of concussion.
7. Anemia is associated with heavy or frequent menstrual cycles and nutritional energy deficit.[1]

The Athlete with Special Needs

The monograph provides an overview of the athlete with special needs and the unique medical issues that will affect their participation in sports. This section reviews the benefits of exercise, methods of evaluation, specific history questions and examination components, functional assessment, diagnostic imaging, and determination of clearance. A history questionnaire and physical examination form are provided in the monograph to assist the provider in this process.[1]

FUTURE DIRECTIONS FOR THE PPE
Need for Further Study and Standardization of the PPE

There is a great need for further research to refine and improve the PPE. The current evidence base for the PPE is limited and is in some respects lacking. The controversy surrounding our current cardiovascular screening process has highlighted this need and brought urgency to this issue. Current research efforts are hindered by the significant variation in the performance of the PPE from state to state. The urgent need of a nationwide standard is greater than ever before.[1]

An electronic version of the PPE

Web-based versions of the PPE hold great promise in the future for improving the process and facilitating standardization of the PPE. Benefits would include: (1) improve efficiency by allowing its completion at home, (2) provide more extensive questions that automatically branch off based on the answers provided, (3) help establish a database to assist in analyzing the effectiveness of each component in the questionnaire, (4) facilitate in the standardization of the PPE, (5) optimize follow-up and medical care for athletes identified with a condition.[1]

SUMMARY

The fourth edition of the *Preparticipation Physical Evaluation* monograph represents the current standard for the performance of the PPE in the United States. With its publication come bold new recommendations to incorporate the PPE into every well-child and adolescent visit as we promote exercise and activity to all children. The ideal setting for the PPE is in the office of the athlete's personal physician to encourage establishment of a medical home for all athletes. The goal of the PPE is to improve the health and safety of athletes in training and competition. However, there is significant controversy regarding the effectiveness of the PPE in reducing the risk of injury or sudden death. Of particular concern is the ability of the PPE to effectively identify athletes at risk for sudden cardiac death.

The Italian national screening system has reported success in reducing the incidence of SCD by using an ECG in addition to a detailed history and physical examination. The American Heart Association consensus panel has recommended against the use of the ECG in the routine screening of athletes. Despite these recommendations, there has been ongoing debate for and against the use of ECG. This ongoing controversy has created an urgency to study the effectiveness of the ECG in a larger

US population of athletes. The lack of a nationwide standard has complicated research efforts because of the significant variation in PPE practices from state to state. The authors, along with the newly formed Campaign and Coalition for Youth Sports Health and Safety, strongly recommend the establishment of a nationwide standard for the PPE. Providing uniformity in the performance of the PPE would improve the care of all young athletes. It would also improve research efforts by allowing meaningful data collection and providing an evidence base to assist in evaluating the effectiveness of the current PPE process. Changes would be based on evidence and outcome data. This uniformity is the best way to make meaningful improvements to the PPE and ultimately improve the health and safety of all young athletes in the United States.

REFERENCES

1. American Academy of Family Physicians, American Academy of Pediatrics, American College of Sports Medicine, et al. Preparticipation Physical Evaluation. In: Roberts W, Bernhardt D, editors. 4th edition. Elk Grove (IL): American Academy of Pediatrics; 2010.
2. Lombardo JA, Badolato SK. The preparticipation physical examination. Clin Cornerstone 2001;3(5):10–24.
3. Glover DW, Maron BJ, Matheson GO. The preparticipation physical examination-steps toward consensus and uniformity. Phys Sportsmed 1999;27(8):29–34.
4. Koester MC. Refocusing the adolescent preparticipation physical evaluation toward preventive health care. J Athl Train 1995;30(4):352–60.
5. Maron BJ, Thompson PD, Puffer JC, et al. Cardiovascular preparticipation screening of competitive athletes: a statement for health professionals from the Sudden Death Committee and Congenital Cardiac Defects committee, American Heart Association. Circulation 1996;94(4):850–6.
6. Maron BJ, Thompson PD, Ackerman MJ, et al. Recommendations and Considerations related to Preparticipation Screening for Cardiovascular Abnormalities in Competitive Athletes: 2007 Update: a scientific statement from the American Heart Association Council on Nutrition, Physical Activity, and Metabolism. Circulation 2007;115:1643–55.
7. Seto CK, Pendleton ME. Preparticipation cardiovascular screening in young athletes: current guidelines and dilemmas. Curr Sports Med Rep 2009;8(2):59–64.
8. Rausch CM, Phillips GC. Adherence to guidelines for cardiovascular screening in current high school preparticipation evaluation forms. J Pediatr 2009;155:584–6.
9. Chang C, McCambride T, Roberts W, et al. Panel endorses preparticipation sports physicals for every child infectious diseases in children. Pediatric Supersite. Available at: http://www.pediatricsupersite.com. Accessed December 15, 2010.
10. Rooks Y, Arvantes J. Youth sports coalition calls for uniform examination process for student athletes. Washington, DC: American Academy of Family Physicians: News Now; 2010.
11. Campbell RM. Preparticipation screening and preparticipation forms. Pacing Clin Electrophysiol 2009;32:S15–8.
12. Corrado D, Basso C, Pavei A, et al. Trends in sudden cardiovascular death in young competitive athletes after implementation of a preparticipation screening program. JAMA 2006;296:1593–601.

13. Drezner J, Berger S, Campbell R. Current controversies in the cardiovascular screening of athletes. Curr Sports Med Rep 2010;9(2):86–92.
14. Maron BJ, Haas TS, Doerer JJ, et al. Comparison of U.S. and Italian experiences with sudden cardiac deaths in young competitive athletes and implications for preparticipation screening strategies. Am J Cardiol 2009;104:276–80.
15. Rao AL, Standaert CJ, Drezner JA, et al. Expert opinion and controversies in musculoskeletal and sports medicine: preventing sudden cardiac death in young athletes. Arch Phys Med Rehabil 2010;91:958–62.

Cardiovascular Screening and the Elite Athlete: Advances, Concepts, Controversies, and a View of the Future

Robert W. Battle, MD[a,b,c,*], Dilaawar J. Mistry, MD, ATC[d],
Rohit Malhotra, MD[c,e], John M. MacKnight, MD[f],
Ethan N. Saliba, PhD, PT, ATC[g,h], Srijoy Mahapatra, BSEE, MD, FHRS[b,c]

KEYWORDS

- Cardiovascular screening • Elite athletes
- Athletic sudden death • Athletic heart
- Hypertrophic cardiomyopathy

For centuries, the elite athlete has enjoyed a status of reverence and adoration in our culture. An early example was the first recognized Olympic Games organized in Greece in 776 BC. The legend of Pheidippedes began with his success as an Olympic champion around 500 BC. Ten years later his celebrated run from the plains of Marathon to Athens to announce the Greek victory over the Persians and his sudden death (SD) that followed marks the beginning of our celebration of the marathon race and has permanently etched athletic SD into our consciousness.[1] The cultural importance of

Conflict of Interest: Dr Srijoy Mahapatra is a consultant to Athletic Heart, LLC and EpiEP.
[a] Department of Medicine, Adult Congenital Heart Clinic, University of Virginia Health System, 1215 Lee Street, PO Box 800158, Charlottesville, VA 22908-0158, USA
[b] University of Virginia Athletic Programs, University of Virginia Health System, PO Box 800158, Charlottesville, VA 22908-0158, USA
[c] Division of Cardiology, University of Virginia Health System, PO Box 800158, Charlottesville, VA 22908-0158, USA
[d] Departments of Athletics and Physical Medicine and Rehabilitation, University of Virginia Health System, 545 Ray C. Hunt Drive, Suite 240, PO Box 801004, Charlottesville, VA 22908-1004, USA
[e] Electrophysiology Fellowship Program, University of Virginia Health System, PO Box 800158, Charlottesville, VA 22908-0158, USA
[f] Department of Medicine, University of Virginia Health System, 415 Ray C. Hunt Drive, Suite 2100, Charlottesville, VA 22908-0671, USA
[g] University of Virginia Health System, 1215 Lee Street, Charlottesville, VA 22908, USA
[h] Department of Athletics, University of Virginia, PO Box 400834, Charlottesville, VA 22904-4834, USA
* Corresponding author.
E-mail address: RWB2FB@hscmail.mcc.virginia.edu

Clin Sports Med 30 (2011) 503–524
doi:10.1016/j.csm.2011.03.001
0278-5919/11/$ – see front matter © 2011 Elsevier Inc. All rights reserved.

the highly trained elite athlete has continued to develop and amplify into modernity. Continuous media coverage on television, radio, Internet, and social networking has elevated the athlete's status to unprecedented heights. Any well-recognized elite athlete participating in sports at the intercollegiate, national team, professional, or Olympic levels occupies an important place in the collective psyche of fellow students, faculty, staff, alumni, and fans around the world. Depending on the athlete and the sport, this effect ripples from thousands to millions of affected individuals. The unexpected death of a young and previously healthy individual from natural causes, although a tragedy for family and friends, is ultimately reconcilable. By contrast, the death of a celebrated athlete, at the summit of their invincibility, extends to countless individuals beyond friends and family. It is generally perceived as somehow preventable and thus it is ultimately irreconcilable. The well-known words of the English poet and scholar A.E. Housman capture the impact of the death of a young athlete on a small town:

> The time you won your town the race
> We chaired you through the market place;
> Man and boy stood cheering by
> And home we brought you shoulder-high.
> Today, the road all runners come,
> Shoulder-high we bring you home,
> And set you at your threshold down,
> Townsman of a stiller town.
>   A.E. Housman (1859–1936): To an Athlete Dying Young

Perhaps the most salient case of athletic SD in the modern era was that of Hank Gathers, who was a senior forward on the Loyola Marymount Division I basketball team in 1990. In the previous season, Gathers had become only the second player in collegiate history to lead the nation in scoring and rebounding.[2] During the 1990 season Loyola Marymount contended for a high national ranking and hoped to gain the national title. Because of the small size of the school and the arc of the team into national consciousness, Loyola Marymount became a favorite of National Collegiate Athletic Association basketball fans across the country. However, events conspired, beginning with Gathers fainting on the court. Both sustained and nonsustained ventricular arrhythmias were documented.[3] Gathers was withdrawn for 3 weeks and treated medically with propranolol. He was not disqualified, returned to competition later in the season, and during a tournament game, Gathers collapsed and died of ventricular fibrillation.

The intricacies of this case, including the probable diagnosis of myocarditis, have been elaborately discussed.[3] The emotional cost to the Gathers family, the Loyola Marymount University family, and the entire sports world is beyond measure. This case also resulted in tremendous financial cost, including an in-court judgment against the physician and an out-of-court settlement with the university. The case of Hank Gathers in 1990 and the tragic timing of those events ushered in a new precedent for those involved in the care and supervision of the elite athlete. Flo Hyman, an Olympic volleyball player with the Marfan syndrome, died 4 years before Gathers and other elite conditioned sports luminaries later suffered similar fates to Gathers, including Pete Maravich, Reggie Lewis, and Jason Collier (basketball), Thomas Herrion (football), Jiri Fischer (hockey), Sergei Grinkov (ice skating), and athletes in Europe and Africa including Marc-Vivian Foe, a soccer player from Cameroon who died of hypertrophic cardiomyopathy (HCM) during a televised international match.[4] Although, the incidence of athletic SD is an uncommon event, the celebrity status of the elite athlete and the consequences of any such catastrophe have generated considerable worldwide interest in cardiovascular screening and programmatic evaluation of athletes to detect unrecognized and potentially life-threatening abnormalities in an effort to reduce this risk to a level as low as can possibly be achieved.

This article addresses programmatic cardiovascular screening and evaluation of the elite athlete at the intercollegiate, national team, professional, and Olympic levels. Although much of the content may apply to high-school and recreational sports at large, it is not specifically designed to address the athletes participating in the vast array of sports activities in today's world.

CONCEPTS AND CONTROVERSY IN CARDIOVASCULAR SCREENING OF THE ELITE ATHLETE

The modern elite athlete is unique to our general population in a myriad of ways. The athlete tests the heart and vascular system to their limit both in training and in competition. The athlete's cardiovascular engine is pushed to the extremes of exertion both in endurance (isotonic, dynamic, or aerobic) and in strength (isometric, static, or anaerobic). The intensity of the performance endured by elite athletes exposes the abnormal cardiovascular system, and any unrecognized underlying weakness could lead to compromised performance, untoward symptoms, and sudden cardiac death. The following can support a strong argument for a comprehensive screening program for elite athletes:

- The occurrence of athletic SD during training or competition is unacceptable. Thus, all reasonable preventative measures should be undertaken.
- Detection of previously undiagnosed arrhythmias, congenital, or acquired heart disease that could affect the health, performance, and longevity of the athlete is of value.
- Detection of autosomal-dominant conditions: HCM, Marfan syndrome and related vascular disorders, long QT, and arrhythmogenic right ventricular cardiomyopathy (ARVC) could lead to evaluation and treatment of siblings and offspring, particularly in families with numerous athletes, who have a 50% chance of being affected.
- The extreme level of performance of elite athletes mandates cardiovascular screening that is not applicable to the general population.
- The prevalent usage of dextroamphetamines and amphetamines to treat attention-deficit/hyperactivity disorder[5] and the widespread availability of these drugs, particularly at the intercollegiate level, mandates knowledge of underlying cardiovascular abnormalities in treated athletes as well as untreated athletes who have unfettered access to these drugs.

The causes of SD in athletes less than the age of 35 years are well known and were established in a landmark paper by Maron and colleagues.[6] HCM, an autosomal-dominant genetic disorder of the cardiac sarcomere, is responsible for 48% of these deaths in the United States. HCM and other congenital cardiac defects account for approximately 80% to 90% of overall deaths, including congenital coronary artery anomalies and diseases of the aorta. Only a few cases were suspected or diagnosed before the athlete's death. There are also many congenital heart conditions and acquired cardiovascular disorders that could affect the future health of the athlete and/or impair performance. Many of these conditions have subtle, if any, physical findings and remain undetected into late adolescence and young adulthood (**Box 1**).

The BAV is of particular importance. This is the most prevalent congenital defect in the general population (2%),[7] especially in males, and may be overlooked because SD as a result of aortic valve disease is rare because the murmurs of significant aortic stenosis (AS) and regurgitation (AR) are easily audible, leading to disease detection and recognition. We encourage renewed attention to the congenital BAV because more than 50% of affected individuals have an associated abnormality of the ascending aorta at the sinuses of Valsalva or above the sinotubular junction. This finding includes asymptomatic young athletes with a functionally normal aortic valve (or mild AS/AR).[8] Furthermore, there is evidence of a significant prevalence of

---

Box 1
Congenital and acquired cardiovascular disorders often undetected in childhood

- Bicuspid aortic valve (BAV): functionally normal or mild valve disorder
  - 50% have associated abnormality of ascending aorta (congenital aortopathy)
- Atrial septal defect (ASD)/left to right shunts
  - Secundum ASD, which includes atrial septal aneurysm with small or multiple ASD/patent foramen ovale
  - Venosus ASD
  - Coronary sinus ASD
  - Partial anomalous pulmonary venous return
- HCM
- Anomalous coronary arteries, coronary artery fistulae
- Marfan syndrome and related disorders
  - Ehlers-Danlos syndrome
  - Loeys-Dietz syndrome
  - MASS phenotype
- Wolff-Parkinson-White syndrome
- Long QT, short QT
- Brugada syndrome
- Ventricular tachycardia, pathologic premature ventricular contractions (PVCs)
- Arrhythmogenic right ventricular cardiomyopathy
- Coarctation of the aorta (particularly milder forms)
- Pulmonary hypertension (particularly mild to moderate forms)
- Myocarditis (acute or with chronically impaired ventricular function)
- Congenital cardiomyopathy (including congenital noncompaction)
- Mitral valve prolapse
- Acquired mild to moderate valvular heart disease: rheumatic, degenerative, radiation-induced, and traumatic (particularly traumatic tricuspid regurgitation)
- Ebstein anomaly
- Congenital absence of the pericardium

ascending aortic dilation in first-degree relatives of patients with BAV, and this aortopathy is not necessarily accompanied by the BAV.[9] It is logical that this may pose a potential risk to young athletes and that detection of these abnormalities would be favorable and would allow for special monitoring of aortic dimensions and disqualification in extreme cases.

The low frequency of SD events in athletes creates a problem inherent to undertaking any screening program.[6,10] Data from the Minneapolis Heart Institute Foundation collected on athletic SD from public records (usually print or broadcast media) document approximately 125 cases of athletic SD per year.[11] Although likely an underestimation of total cases of SD because of underreporting, this statistic may capture most cases of elite athlete SD. Broad-based testing of a large population with a low incidence of events creates the difficult epidemiologic problem of testing results containing more false-positive results than true-positive results. If screening errors for each athlete who has a true abnormality sideline several healthy athletes with normal cardiovascular systems, then clearly our screening protocol has failed.

Accordingly, any comprehensive screening program for elite athletes should be structured to maximize true-positive results and minimize false-positive results. The remaining sections of this article review past and current testing strategies and explore new testing strategies that could improve diagnostic yield and reduce unwanted false-positive results.

CARDIOVASCULAR SCREENING OF THE ELITE ATHLETE

Standards and guidelines for programs and individual health care providers involved in athletic cardiovascular screening are lacking, as are credentialing and recommendations for knowledgeable caregivers in this area. In practice, subspecialty health care providers with little practical experience may evaluate athletes and associated cardiovascular diagnostic studies with athletes, including the spectrum of the athlete's heart. Furthermore, providers may have limited knowledge and exposure to congenital heart disease, HCM, arrhythmogenic right ventricular dysplasia, long QT, and anomalous coronary arteries. Practices vary from state to state and it is fair to assume the current system of screening is not ideally designed to maximize the yield of true-positive results in this population and simultaneously minimize undesirable false-positive results.

History and Physical Examination: Initiating the Process

Ideally, the initial history and physical examination should be performed within a credentialed sports medicine facility. This strategy ensures the vital association of the athlete to a licensed sports medicine provider and connects the athlete to a medical home to begin a relationship between the athlete and provider that promotes trust and full disclosure of symptoms and past history from the athlete. The primary sports medicine provider, in turn, navigates the subspecialty referral process, including cardiovascular screening, supports the athlete, and integrates the medical plan in concert with sophisticated sports training staff. It is essential that the medical home of the athlete fully integrates the athletic training staff who have developed a sophisticated involvement in the complete health of athletes, with a wide array of knowledge and technology, including stethoscopes, blood pressure cuffs, and automatic external defibrillators. Athletic trainers also take an active role in coordinating medical appointments for athletes, and attending those appointments allows the athletic trainer to carry the medical information back to the athletic arena. This valuable resource can assist in execution of the plan; report on the consequences of the plan; and provide on-site eyes and ears that greatly assist in management and diagnosis of cardiovascular disorders.

The history and physical examination includes screening for a family history of SD or heart disease in relatives less than 50 years old, a detailed personal history, and physical examination. This strategy has been described in detail by Maron and colleagues[12] and was adopted by the American Heart Association consensus panel recommendations for preparticipation screening.[13] The history and physical examination are limited and cannot be expected to detect most dangerous cardiovascular diseases. In a retrospective analysis, only 3% of athletes who suffered SD and had participated in screening history and physical examination were considered to have possible cardiovascular abnormalities, and none was disqualified.[14]

The physical examination is likely to be helpful in screening patients with the Marfan syndrome and related vascular disorders (Loeys-Dietz syndrome[15] and Ehlers-Danlos syndrome), with careful attention paid to skin (laxity, striae) the musculoskeletal system (arachnodactyly, scoliosis, anterior chest wall deformity), eyes (myopia, ectopia lentis), and general assessment for any syndromic abnormalities (bifid uvula, cleft palate, hypertelorism, micrognathia). Detection of these disorders is critical because aortic dissection, although often not fatal, changes the remainder of that individual's life (**Fig. 1**). Careful auscultation of the heart is important and the systolic opening click of the functionally normal BAV can be subtle and should not be overlooked. In general, the physical examination may prove to be of greater value as sports medicine continues to grow and experienced evaluators become more prevalent.

Family history is important but also limited. For example, Marfan syndrome and HCM are complex genetic disorders and up to 25% to 33% of individuals affected have spontaneous mutations that are new and private. Thus, a negative family history is misleading.[16,17] Any family history of SD before the age of 35 years mandates a referral to cardiology to determine what further diagnostic testing is indicated because of the prevalent genetic transmission of HCM, long QT, ARVC, and Marfan syndrome and related vascular disorders (including familial BAV/congenital aortopathy).

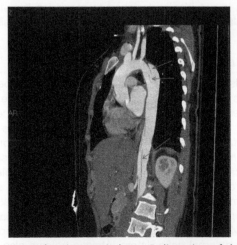

Fig. 1. CT scan with contrast showing a spiral type B dissection of the descending thoracic aorta (*arrows* indicate the intimal flap) in a female intercollegiate swimmer with the Marfan syndrome. The dissection occurred during practice. The sinuses of Valsalva were only borderline abnormal with an eccentric posterior sinus.

Diagnostic Testing

Routine diagnostic testing beyond the history and physical examination is controversial and not widely agreed on or standardized. Additional noninvasive testing strategies might include electrocardiography (ECG), transthoracic echocardiography (TTE), exercise testing (ETT), Holter or event recording, genetic testing, computed tomography (CT) angiography, and cardiac magnetic resonance imaging (CMR) with or without contrast.

For the purpose of screening, we believe that only tests that are noninvasive and pose no potential health threat to the athlete are acceptable. Accordingly, radiation (CT) and administration of intravenous contrast (CT and CMR) are unacceptable tools and should be used only when a significant disorder is suspected. Genetic testing for conditions like long QT, HCM, Marfan syndrome, and related disorders should be performed only by experienced providers under select circumstances. For the most part recognition and treatment of these disorders is clinical. Genetic testing is expensive and limited because a negative test does not exclude the condition being tested and a positive test does not always well predict the phenotypic expression of that condition within the individual of concern.

The 2 most widely used tests are the ECG and TTE and these are discussed separately. Routine use of ETT to screen young elite athletes is not of value because of the low incidence of coronary artery disease and because ETT is inconsistent and not generally helpful in detecting anomalous coronary artery variations that have been associated with SD.[18] Selective use of ETT may be of value in symptomatic athletes with exercise-induced arrhythmias. Of particular concern is catecholaminergic polymorphic ventricular tachycardia (CPVT), which is a genetic disorder that can lead to SD. ETT may also benefit older athletes with risk factors present that could increase the risk of premature coronary artery disease.

In athletes more than the age of 35 years, the leading cause of SD shifts away from HCM and overwhelmingly favors coronary artery disease (80%).[3] To reiterate, it is essential that the subspecialty cardiovascular professionals who are involved in any screening program and perform and interpret further diagnostic testing have a thorough understanding of the normal range of physiologic adaptations that comprise the athlete's heart[19] and also have experience with arrhythmias as well as a variety of conditions present in the population of adults with congenital heart disease. Otherwise, athletes with normal adaptations are sidelined unnecessarily and those with real cardiovascular issues may be underdiagnosed.

ECG

ECG is a safe, relatively inexpensive, and routinely available screening tool for the elite athlete and can provide useful diagnostic information about underlying electrical or structural abnormalities of the heart that could place the athlete at risk. Accordingly, the ECG has been the most widely used cardiovascular diagnostic test in athletic screening. However, this is a complicated diagnostic and interpretive process because most elite athletes manifest some degree of electrocardiographic aberration when compared with the normal population because of intense athletic training, which leads to important alterations in both structure and autonomic regulation of the heart.[20-28] Most highly trained athletes have an abnormal resting ECG with well-documented training-related abnormalities, including sinus bradycardia, first-degree atrioventricular block, complete right bundle branch block (RBBB), early repolarization, and QRS voltage criteria for left ventricular hypertrophy (LVH). LVH poses a particular problem in the athlete because it may simply reflect the physiologic adaptation to isometric training (LVH), or isotonic training (dilation with increased LV mass), or a combination of the two. The challenge for any screening program is to differentiate between this adaptive response and the pathologic condition of HCM.

Several factors influence the type and degree of electrocardiographic abnormalities in the elite athlete. Physiologic and structural changes that alter the ECG are more common in males and in athletes of African or Caribbean descent.[29–31] The type of training undertaken by the athlete is also important, with physiologic abnormalities detected on ECG more common in endurance sports that also include significant amounts of static/isometric training, such as cycling, rowing, canoeing, and cross-country skiing.[29] More recent data including sports prevalent in the United States suggest that ECG abnormalities are also more common in football.[30] Race can accentuate this as well, with male black football players twice as likely to have ECG abnormalities as their white counterparts.[30] Angiotensin gene polymorphisms may also predispose athletes to abnormal remodeling and thus more extensive increases in LV mass and wall thickness.[32,33] Cardiovascular screening inclusive of ECG poses a more difficult interpretive challenge in the male athlete compared with the female athlete because female athletes are more likely to have a normal or only mildly abnormal ECG.[29] Race affects the female athlete's ECG in a fashion similar to that noted with males but the differences are less dramatic.[34]

Corrado and colleagues[28] published findings of a 25-year experience with elite Italian athletes participating in a wide array of sports. This study has helped to establish thorough guidelines for the interpretation of ECG in elite athletes. It also provides the modern screening process with the sophistication to discern the difference between physiologic adaptation and potentially dangerous electrophysiologic or structural abnormalities. From the Italian perspective this strategy has been shown to be cost-effective.[35] Corrado and colleagues[28] have also provided insights regarding the types of abnormalities that are "uncommon and training un-related ECG changes," including T-wave inversion, ST segment depression, pathologic q waves, left atrial enlargement, left axis deviation/left anterior hemiblock, right axis deviation/left posterior hemiblock, right ventricular hypertrophy, ventricular preexcitation (Wolff-Parkinson-White), complete left bundle branch block (LBBB) and RBBB, long or short QT, and Brugada-like early repolarization. LVH by voltage criteria is a common ECG abnormality in athletes, reflecting increases in LV wall thickness or mass. This physiologic adaptation usually results in increased QRS amplitude alone, not in combination with ST segment depression, T-wave inversion, or prolongation of the QRS or shift in QRS axis.[24–26,28,29,35–40] In the elite athlete these changes are adaptations in hypertrophy and mass and usually do not correlate with underlying HCM on TTE. However, caution is advised because the sensitivity of a negative ECG in the detection of HCM is limited by the 20% of individuals with HCM who have normal or only mildly abnormal ECG.[41] Simply stated, ECG alone does not uncover all individuals with HCM.

ARVC has historically been a difficult clinical diagnosis but more recently criteria for diagnosis by CMR have become more specific.[42] ECG may reveal T-wave inversion of greater than 2mm in 2 or more adjacent leads (a finding uncommon in older athletes) and this finding may warrant magnetic resonance imaging (MRI) screening for ARVC if TTE reveals no evidence of other structural heart disease.[28,43,44] Examples of abnormal screening ECG are provided in **Figs. 2–6**.

The complexity of this interpretive process has understandably created controversy with regard to mandated ECG screening of athletes. In the United States, use of ECG in screening has been advocated,[45] and the limitations and pitfalls inherent in widespread screening have also been elaborately argued.[46] Mandated preparticipation

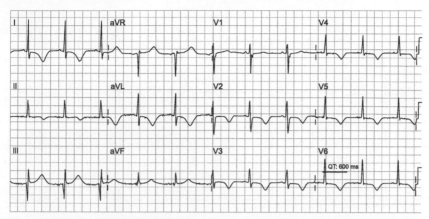

Fig. 2. Long QT in a patient with torsades de pointes. The QT interval indicated by the bar in V6 is prolonged to approximately 600 ms.

ECG screening has been discouraged[46,47] and has not been endorsed by the American College of Cardiology, the American Heart Association, and most recently in 2005 at the 36th Bethesda Conference on Eligibility Recommendations for Competitive Athletes with Cardiovascular Disorders.[12,13] For the past 27 years there has been an Atlantic divide on this subject, with the Italian experience including a federally subsidized preparticipation screening program inclusive of ECG in all athletes.[48,49] Italian investigators have published observations suggesting a reduction in the overall rate of athletic SD after implementation of this more aggressive strategy and further argue that preparticipation screening with ECG led to the identification and disqualification of athletes with HCM and as a result, the demographics of athletic SD in the Veneto region of Italy have shifted away from HCM as the most common cause of SD and toward ARVC.[50] In this last study of 269 pathologic cases of athletic SD only 1 athlete had HCM, with more cases attributable to ARVC (22%).[50]

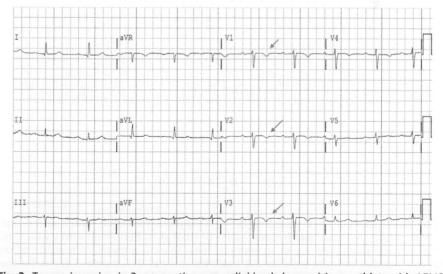

Fig. 3. T-wave inversion in 3 consecutive precordial leads (*arrows*) in an athlete with ARVC.

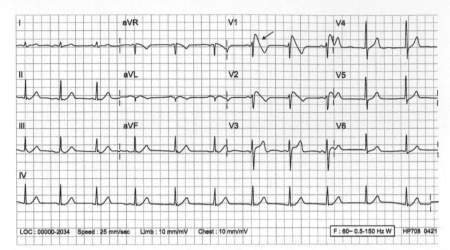

Fig. 4. Brugada syndrome with coved type ST segment elevation greater than 2 mm in V1 (*arrow*) followed by a negative/inverted T wave.

There will be continued controversy regarding the implementation of any complex interpretive process like ECG screening and we believe there is merit on both sides of the argument. In order for the benefit to exceed the harm and for any program to be cost-effective, it must be advanced in a sophisticated manner with knowledgeable providers involved at all levels. Although one can argue that the Italian system has merit and should be emulated, it can also be argued that logistically we are not ready, capable, nor can we afford implementation of widespread ECG screening of elite athletes in the United States.[46]

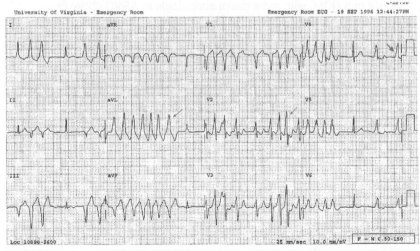

Fig. 5. Wolff-Parkinson-White syndrome. During sinus rhythm the delta wave is seen in lead V4 (*thick arrow*). There are also frequent salvos of rapid atrial fibrillation with a wide QRS, which indicates conduction via an accessory pathway (*narrow arrows*). With atrial fibrillation conducted at this rate (close to 300 beats per minute) this athlete is at risk for the degeneration of the rhythm to ventricular fibrillation and thus SD.

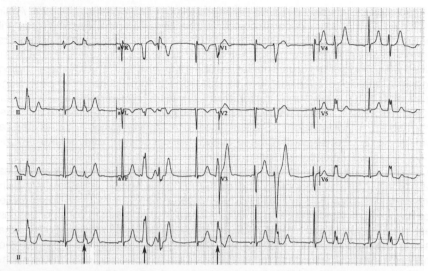

Fig. 6. A 17-year-old female Division I collegiate pole-vaulter with PVCs on screening ECG. ETT revealed polymorphic ventricular foci (*arrows*). Epinephrine challenge corroborated the diagnosis of CPVT. This athlete was disqualified and the arrhythmia was suppressed with a β-blocker.

TTE

The debate over inclusion of TTE in athletic preparticipation screening is even more complex, and there are no guidelines in Europe or the United States endorsing routine use of TTE unless the history, physical examination, family history, or screening ECG warrants further testing. Much as with ECG, TTE has historically struggled to define normal with regard to physiologic versus pathologic hypertrophy. This process remains challenging and controversial, but great progress in this area has been made and with astute analysis the gray zone between normal adaptation to training and abnormal physiology has been clarified, giving us sharper and more powerful clinical tools to separate the two.[4,51,52]

The phenotypic expression of the pathologic condition of HCM is highly variable, with affected genotypes manifesting LV wall thickness ranging from normal (<12 mm) to mild to moderate hypertrophy (13–15 mm) to severe (30–50 mm).[4,17,53] Normal physiologic adaptation to training frequently shows increases in LV wall thickness into the upper limit of normal and in some cases LV wall thickness extends into the gray zone of 13 to 15 mm.[52,54] This finding characterizes the problem of overlap between the elite athlete and the spectrum of HCM, with cases disguised and difficult to recognize coming from both groups.

However, there are several features that careful echocardiographic analysis can assess to help unravel this complex overlap and separate normal adaptation from HCM. LV end-diastolic cavity dimensions of greater than 55 mm are common in trained athletes but rare in HCM. The LV cavity in HCM is usually small and dilation rarely occurs in the context of late-stage systolic dysfunction and progression to dilated cardiomyopathy.[4,55] Systolic anterior motion (SAM) of the anterior leaflet of the mitral valve, although definitively part of the HCM spectrum, is not a feature of the athlete's heart.[4] SAM typically occurs with small LV cavity size and would be unlikely in an athlete whose training included significant amounts of isotonic/dynamic exercise, with those effects of volume loading leading to a larger than normal cavity size. Again, this finding is not absolute because one could conceive of a scenario in which primarily isometric/static training could lead to hypertrophy and in the proper setting of dehydration could lead to SAM associated with smaller LV cavity size. Diastolic abnormalities of pulsed wave Doppler or tissue Doppler are absent in athletes,[56,57] thus these findings suggest a pathologic condition such as HCM or restrictive/constrictive physiology. Areas of regional hypertrophy rather than concentric hypertrophy are also more suggestive of HCM. This is 1 area in which CMR has been shown to have greater sensitivity than TTE.[58–60] Usage of TTE as a diagnostic tool to assess this complex area can be enhanced but if screening TTE is too limited then our ability to differentiate may also be compromised within the screening process.

Gender and race continue to be important in screening TTE. Female athletes are less likely to have LV cavity dilation, and of the 600 elite female athletes undergoing screening TTE, none had LV wall thickness greater than 12 mm.[61] As noted earlier, race has a more limited impact on females but remains important to consider because black female athletes had LV wall thickness measurements 0.6 mm greater than their white female counterparts.[34] Accordingly, the gray zone problem is more common among male elite athletes than female, and an astute screening echocardiographer would be concerned that LV wall thickness of greater than 12 mm associated with normal or small cavity size in a female athlete likely represents HCM.[4] Examples of athletic heart and HCM are shown in **Fig. 7**.

CMR performed with gadolinium can detect fibrosis of the heart within the spectrum of HCM and late gadolinium enhancement (LGE) may also have important prognostic value (**Fig. 8**).[62,63] There are cases that are difficult and perhaps impossible to resolve and it is prudent to reevaluate all athletes diagnosed by screening with pathologic hypertrophy or HCM after detraining to reassess wall thickness and determine if the hypertrophy persists or regresses. CMR can be of diagnostic value to assess acute myocarditis or persistent sequelae of myocarditis that could pose long-term risk to the athlete (**Fig. 9**). Genetic testing has a limited role and can only confirm a positive mutation; a negative test does not exclude HCM because of the frequency of spontaneous and yet undetected mutations.

The congenital anomalous coronary artery is responsible for a significant remaining percentage of athletic SD (14%),[6] particularly the left coronary artery arising from the right sinus, with fewer cases involving the right coronary arising from the left sinus.[18] This anomaly escapes detection by traditional screening methods in the United States because only a few have premonitory symptoms and of those all (9/9) had a normal ECG and, when performed, stress ECG with maximal exercise was also normal (6/6).[18] The only safe and noninvasive opportunity to diagnose this anomaly in preparticipation screening is TTE, which can identify the right and left coronary arteries in most elite athletes (95%).[64] However, recognition of abnormal coronary anomalies is another matter and in the practical context, coronary origins and courses are not routinely assessed in most adult echo laboratories. Accordingly, routine and broad-based screening using sonographers with limited experience with normal coronaries and even less experience with anomalous coronary arteries seems an inadequate solution to this difficult problem. By contrast, coronary origins and courses are routinely assessed in congenital echo laboratories because of the frequent occurrence of anomalous coronary arteries within the spectrum of congenital heart disease. Because both CMR and CT angiography are expensive and require contrast intravenously for definitive anatomic clarification, we believe that a careful congenital approach to TTE may be the only hope of having any impact with successful screening for this disorder.

TTE easily detects dilation of the ascending aorta at the sinuses of Valsalva, which could herald dissection or rupture in undetected Marfan syndrome or related diseases

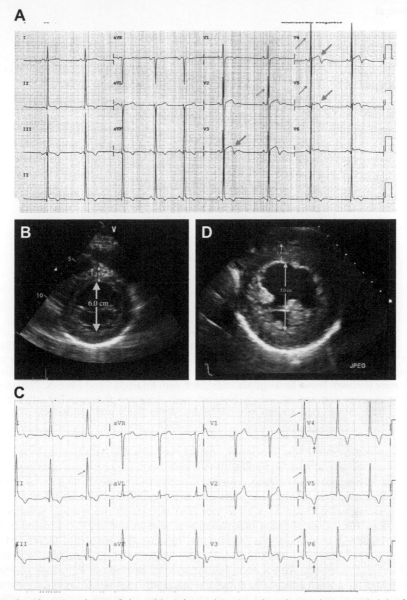

Fig. 7. (A–D) ECG and TTE of the athletic heart (Fig. 7A, B) and HCM (Fig. 7C, D). (A) African American Division I basketball player. ECG shows diffusely increased QRS voltage without QRS widening (*narrow arrows*) and upwardly convex ST elevation followed by inverted T waves (*broad arrows*). This ECG shows the more pronounced abnormalities of the athletic heart seen in African American athletes. (B) This same athlete's short-axis TTE image shows a mild increase in septal wall thickness to 1.25 cm (*narrow arrows*) with mild LV cavity dilation of 6.0 cm (*broad arrows*) and a corresponding increase in LV mass. This is a representative example of athlete's heart in an elite African American athlete. (C) An 18-year-old high-school football player with HCM. The ECG reveals increased QRS voltage but with mild prolongation in QRS duration (*narrow arrows*) and prominent T-wave inversion (*broad arrows*). (D) Short-axis image of a TTE in an African American Division I basketball player with HCM and exertional angina. The septum is abnormally hypertrophied, measuring 1.6 cm (*narrow arrows*) and the LV cavity size is 5.0 cm, which is considerably smaller than noted with the athletic heart. Stress echocardiography revealed complete systolic LV cavity obliteration.

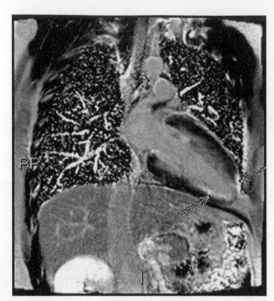

Fig. 8. Cardiac MRI of an 18-year-old high-school football player with HCM (this athlete's ECG is shown in **Fig. 7C**). There is subendocardial LGE involving the inferior wall in both the mid and apical part of the left ventricle as well as delayed transmural enhancement of the apex (*arrows*). These findings are consistent with infarction and fibrosis. This athlete was also experiencing angina, which resolved with β-blocker therapy. The athlete was removed from competition and an internal cardiac defibrillator was implanted.

of the vascular system. The aortopathy associated with the BAV occurs in approximately 50% of all patients, including those with functionally normal and minimally abnormal valves that easily evade detection. At the University of Virginia, screening echocardiography has detected 3 male athletes with BAV of 854 athletes and one has an associated aortopathy with a root that is mild to moderately enlarged at 4.4 cm (**Fig. 10**). None of these diagnoses was known before TTE screening. The BAV aortopathy can involve the sinuses of Valsalva but also can isolate to the ascending aorta above the sinotubular junction, which can be overlooked with standard adult TTE imaging. With a complete congenital protocol it is routine to image this aspect of the aorta 1 interspace above the standard long-axis sinus view and rotate the transducer clockwise toward the short-axis view to ideally image this difficult anatomic area. Additional attention to the transverse arch and descending thoracic aorta from suprasternal views coupled with detailed subcostal imaging of the abdominal aorta provides additional diagnostic accuracy in forms of mild coarctation and other vascular disorders that affect the aorta remote from the sinuses of Valsalva.

Focused congenital imaging can also detect a host of other previously undetected conditions, as noted earlier (see **Box 1**). Although most are not life threatening, altered physiology could affect performance and lead to exercise-related symptoms of cardiovascular compromise.

CARDIOVASCULAR SCREENING IN THE ELITE ATHLETE: OUR VIEW OF THE FUTURE

Sports medicine and sports training have become increasingly more sophisticated, providing comprehensive care for all aspects of the athlete's health. This is the

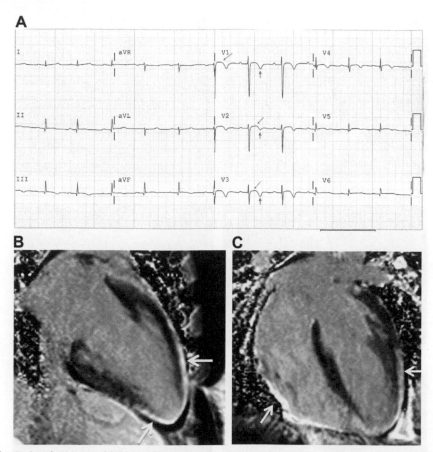

Fig. 9. (A–C) 21-year-old African American Division I college basketball player with myocarditis. This athlete initially presented with syncope and had a second syncopal episode 5 months later. (A) ECG reveals persistent diffuse ST segment elevation (*narrow arrows*) followed by T-wave inversion (*broader arrows*). (B) Cardiac MRI shows LGE of the epicardial aspect of the anteroapex and inferoapex (*arrows*). (C) Late epicardial enhancement of the right ventricular free wall is also noted (*leftward arrow*). The ECG is suggestive of chronic pericarditis and myocarditis, and the typical MRI finding of epicardial LGE is characteristic of this disorder compared with the patchy LGE/fibrosis seen in HCM. Electrophysiologic study revealed easily inducible rapid ventricular tachycardia, and the athlete is currently restricted from competition.

foundation of the medical home of the athlete and the subspecialty care of elite athletes with known or suspected abnormalities must follow this initiative, with providers experienced in the complex interplay between normal physiologic adaptation and pathologic conditions. Our current status with the cardiovascular care of elite athletes in many ways mirrors the problem facing the adult congenital heart disease (ACHD) population 20 years ago. It was widely recognized that a large population of patients was emerging with a unique variety of care issues without a sufficient workforce of knowledgeable providers available regionally to ensure the best possible care.[65] It would be of great benefit to all elite athletes if centers of care including expertise in screening and evaluation of athletes could be developed regionally (similar to the programs currently developed for adults with congenital heart disease) to provide

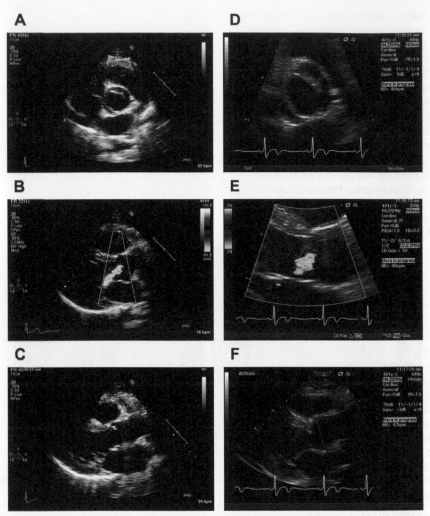

Fig. 10. (*A–F*) TTE examples of a familial BAV syndrome in 2 brothers, both of whom are Division I lacrosse players, and one of whom has an associated congenital aortopathy. (*A*) Parasternal short-axis view of an 18-year-old athlete with a BAV (*arrows*) with fusion of the right and left coronary cusps and a horizontally oblique aperture. (*B*) Parasternal long-axis view with color Doppler showing moderate aortic insufficiency (AR) oriented directly toward the anterior leaflet of the mitral valve (*arrow*). This posterior orientation of AR is characteristic of prolapse of the anterior cusp. (*C*) Parasternal long-axis view showing the typical systolic doming of the aortic cusps (*arrow*) and measurement of the ascending aorta at the sinuses of Valsalva is normal for body surface area at 3.4 cm (*red line bordered by x's*). (*D*) Parasternal short-axis view of 21-year-old brother with a near identical valve with the same fusion pattern and aperture (*arrows*). (*E*) Parasternal long-axis view showing a similar orientation of the AR by color Doppler (*arrow*). In this brother the AR is mild to moderate. (*F*) Parasternal long-axis view showing the presence of a congenital aortopathy in the older brother. Maximal dilation is mild to moderate at 4.4 cm when measured at the sinuses of Valsalva (*red line bordered by x's*). Both brothers are eligible to play based on current guidelines.[13] Because of the hemodynamic effects of elite training that could accelerate either the AR or the aortopathy, both athletes are being evaluated by TTE every 6 months.

colleges, universities, and national and professional teams with referral options for thorough and experienced evaluations.

One can easily envision that larger universities particularly at the Division I level are in a good position to develop this expertise and establish programs, with the primary mission being the cardiovascular health and well-being of the athlete with secondary but important goals of physician training and research. Providers with a broader experience in screening are in the best position to interpret screening diagnostic studies and to guide the athlete through any further diagnostic testing. The relationship of the physician provider and the athlete has received particular attention because of potential personal, ethical, legal, or institutional conflicts of interest.[66,67] Although these conflicts can never be fully resolved, in general the physician should be committed first to the health and safety of the athlete and simultaneously balance the responsibility toward the school or team responsible for the athlete.

Mandated screening currently performed in Italy enjoys the financial support of the Italian government and backing within Italian law. This strategy is not feasible in the United States, where, for example, screening colonoscopy or breast mammography is recommended but not mandated. Instead, the type of program and the choices of diagnostic testing are largely decided by the schools and teams that host the athletes. We believe that institutions responsible for the well-being of elite athletes are likely to have significant motivation to protect their athletes from any serious adverse event. Future screening and ongoing care programs can learn from the large body of work in this area to develop a more precise set of tools initiated at the moment of contact with the athlete. Because of the developed depth of our understanding, both ECG and TTE are useful and appropriate diagnostic tools for cardiovascular screening of elite athletes.

ECG is useful in the diagnosis of both electrical and structural abnormalities of the heart. However, ECG is inherently compromised by lack of sensitivity and specificity, particularly in the detection of structural heart disease. There is considerable overlap between physiologic and pathologic hypertrophy, and ECG cannot detect abnormalities of the aorta or anomalous coronary artery, and may also be unrevealing in a host of congenital and acquired conditions that could be dangerous or compromise performance. For these reasons we believe that both ECG and TTE should be used together to enhance diagnostic yield and reduce the rate of false-positive results that could interrupt training and participation unnecessarily.

Inclusion of TTE into routine cardiovascular screening requires providers and sonographers with expertise in athlete's heart and congenital heart disease. We advocate a more congenital approach to TTE screening, with more focus on the aorta (ascending, arch, descending thoracic, and abdominal), coronary arteries, atrial septum, and attention to the possibility of regional (especially apical) hypertrophy. This recommendation supplements standard views with more subcostal and suprasternal imaging. We include standard TTE long-axis and short-axis views, and apical 4-chamber and 2-chamber views with careful measurement of LV wall thickness and mass. All valves and great arteries are subject to pulsed, continuous, and color Doppler. This strategy includes calculation of pulmonary artery and right atrial pressure. Tissue Doppler is performed if there is LVH, any question of HCM, or left atrial enlargement. Our early experience indicates that this assessment can be accomplished in less than 8 minutes and with progressive experience the duration required will likely decrease. Although they are noble in intention and common in practice, a word of caution is due regarding screening programs with limited TTE that do not record images.[68] This practice does not allow for retrospective analysis of data, later analysis off-line, and, if a death were to occur, this could create legal vulnerability as a result of the act of screening with no reviewable data. Whether our recommended approach to screening in this manner improves the positive yield of diagnostic testing and simultaneously reduces the rate of false-positive results remains to be seen. We are not aware of previous studies that have favored a more congenital approach to this problem.

If we can follow the lead of the regional programs in ACHD with similar regional programs developed for elite athletes, then a safe medical home will have been created. A reliable network can be established through trainers and athletic departments to market these programs and develop consultation for any athlete within the region. For example, at the University of Virginia there are approximately 700 collegiate athletes. In the remainder of the Commonwealth of Virginia there are more than 100 colleges and universities, with thousands of elite athletes. Those athletes suspected of cardiovascular abnormalities require additional testing including TTE, ETT, CMR/CT angiography, Holter and event monitoring, and electrophysiologic studies. Because most athletes are fully insured, financial models outlining success that are fiscally sustainable may qualify for other sources of internal or external funding that can support these programs. The success of this type of program could lead to more widespread and affordable screening expertise for neighboring institutions and athletes.

The future of cardiovascular ultrasonography (TTE) is rapidly moving toward a less expensive and more widely available technology. Portable laptop-sized echo machines are available at 25% of the cost of larger hospital-based machines. These machines are available for approximately $60,000, and image and data quality are sufficient for these purposes. The next generation is evolving further, with echo capability now available in a size slightly larger than a smart phone for approximately $8000. Accordingly, future screening packages could be offered at a fraction of previously incurred cost. However, caution is encouraged, particularly in the realm of echocardiography, because unlike ECG, TTE is acquired with dynamic imaging and is highly dependent on the skill and experience of both the ultrasonography technician and the interpreting cardiologist. A dynamic interaction between the two produces the most desirable results.

Potential sources of future cardiovascular providers in this area could easily draw from 2 important sources. The first source could come from the large pool of former and current athletes within the realm of the cardiovascular subspecialty. There would be increased job satisfaction among provider athletes motivated to remain involved in sports. It is clear in our program that athletes prefer their providers to have an athletic background. Although meeting this preference is clearly not required, athletes are more comfortable if the unique aspects of their existence are more completely understood. The second source could emerge from providers with expertise in the care of adults with congenital heart disease. These providers have the most extensive experience with the structural conditions likely to be encountered in the athlete, and this new clinical opportunity could provide an exciting and new supplement to their current practice, which, in many cases, is not enough to sustain full-time support of clinical staff.

We see this situation as a unique and exciting opportunity for providers. Athletes are a highly motivated and engaging population. All involved in the program at the University of Virginia find our participation with the athletes to be an energy source, rather than energy sink. We strive toward a 24-hour turnaround for athletes of concern to be evaluated so that training and participation are not interrupted by unnecessary delays. Our program is comprised of sports medicine staff, a wide array of athletic training staff, 5 cardiologists (areas of expertise include ACHD, electrophysiology, and pediatric cardiology), 1 cardiology nurse, and 2 congenital sonographers. Four senior cardiovascular fellows participate in screening, clinical evaluations, grant proposals, and clinical research. Thus far the enthusiasm to participate has exceeded our ability to accommodate all who would like to be involved. If this article inspires new involvement and the development of new ideas and programs for our athletes then our goals will have been fulfilled.

REFERENCES

1. Sweet WE. Sport and recreation in ancient Greece. New York: Oxford University Press; 1987.
2. Pond M, editor. Official 1990 NCAA basketball records. Overland Park (KS): NCAA; 1991. p. 152–3.
3. Maron B. Sudden death in young athletes: lessons from the Hank Gathers affair. N Engl J Med 1993;329:55–7.
4. Maron BJ. Distinguishing hypertrophic cardiomyopathy from athlete's heart physiological remodeling: clinical significance, diagnostic strategies and implications for pre-participation screening. Br J Sports Med 2009;43:649–66.
5. Hicky G, Fricker P. Attention deficit hyperactivity disorder, CNS stimulants and sport. Sports Med 1999;27(1):11–21.
6. Maron BJ, Epstein SE, Roberts WC. Causes of sudden death in competitive athletes. J Am Coll Cardiol 1986;7:204–14.
7. Roberts WC. The congenitally bicuspid aortic valve: a study of 85 autopsy cases. Am J Cardiol 1970;26:72.
8. Nitri S, Sorbo MD, Mari M, et al. Aortic root dilation in young men with normally functioning bicuspid aortic valves. Heart 1999;82:19.
9. Biner S, Rafique AM, Ray I, et al. Aortopathy is prevalent in relatives of bicuspid aortic valve patients. J Am Coll Cardiol 2009;53:2288–95.
10. Maron BJ, Gohman TE, Aeppli D. Prevalence of sudden cardiac death during competitive sports activities in Minnesota high school athletes. J Am Coll Cardiol 1998;32:1991–4.
11. Frieldewald VE, Maron BJ, Roberts WC. The editor's round table: sudden cardiac death in athletes. Am J Cardiol 2007;100:1451–9.
12. Maron BJ, Thompson PD, Puffer JC, et al. Cardiovascular participating screening of competitive athletes. A statement for health professionals from the Sudden Death Committee (clinical cardiology) and Congenital Cardiac Defects Committee (cardiovascular disease in the young), American Heart Association. Circulation 1996;94:850–6.
13. Maron BT, Douglas PS, Graham TP, et al. Task Force 1: preparticipation screening and diagnosis of cardiovascular disease in athletes. 36th Bethesda conference: eligibility recommendations for competitive athletes with cardiovascular abnormalities. Circulation 2005;85:1322–6.
14. Maron BJ, Shirani J, Poliac LC, et al. Sudden death in young competitive athletes: clinical demographic and pathological profiles. JAMA 1996;276:199–204.
15. Loeys BL, Schwarze U, Holm T, et al. Aneurysm syndromes caused by mutations in the TGF-beta receptor. N Engl J Med 2006;355:788–98.
16. Pyeritz RE. The Marfan syndrome in childhood: features, natural history and differential diagnosis. Prog Pediatr Cardiol 1996;5:151–7.
17. Maron BJ, McKenna WJ, Danielson GK, et al. American College of Cardiology/European Society of Cardiology clinical expert consensus document on hypertrophic cardiomyopathy. J Am Coll Cardiol 2003;42:1687–713.
18. Basso C, Maron BJ, Corrado D, et al. Clinical profile of the congenital coronary anomalies with origin from wrong aortic sinus leading to sudden death in young competitive athletes. J Am Coll Cardiol 2000;35:1493–501.

19. Pluim BM, Zwinderman AH, Van der Laarse A, et al. The athlete's heart: a meta-analysis of cardiac structure and function. Circulation 2000;101:336–44.
20. Huston P, Puffer JC, MacMillian RW. The athletic heart syndrome. N Engl J Med 1985;315:24–32.
21. Fagard R. Athlete's heart. Heart 2003;89:1455–61.
22. Oakley CM. The electrocardiogram in the highly trained athlete. Cardiol Clin 1992;10:295–302.
23. Barbier J, Ville N, Kervio K, et al. Sports-specific features of athlete's heart and their relation to echocardiographic parameters. Herz 2006;31:531–43.
24. Bjornstad H, Storstein L, Meen HD, et al. Electrocardiographic findings in athletic students and controls. Cardiology 1992;79:290–305.
25. Storstein L, Bjornstad H, Hals O, et al. Electrocardiographic findings according to sex in athletes and controls. Cardiology 1991;79:227–36.
26. Bjornstad H, Storstein L, Dyre Meen H, et al. Electrocardiographic findings according to level of fitness and sport activity. Cardiology 1993;83:268–79.
27. Bjornstad H, Storstein L, Meen HD, et al. Electrocardiographic findings of repolarization in athletic students and control subjects. Cardiology 1994;84: 51–60.
28. Corrado D, Pelliccia A, Heidbuchel H, et al. Recommendations for interpretation of the 12-lead electrocardiogram in the athlete. Eur Heart J 2010;31:243–59.
29. Pellicia A, Maron BJ, Culasso F, et al. Clinical significance of abnormal electrocardiographic patterns in trained athletes. Circulation 2000;102:278–84.
30. Magalaski A, Maron BJ, Main ML, et al. Relation of race to electrocardiographic patterns in elite American football players. J Am Coll Cardiol 2008;51:2250–5.
31. Basavarajaiah S, Boraita A, Whyte G, et al. Ethnic differences in left ventricular remodeling in highly-trained athletes: relevance to differentiating physiologic left ventricular hypertrophy from hypertrophic cardiomyopathy. J Am Coll Cardiol 2008;51:2256–62.
32. Montgomery HE, Clarkson P, Dollery CM, et al. Association of angiotension-converting enzyme gene I/D polymorphism with change in left ventricular mass in response to physical training. Circulation 1997;96:741–7.
33. Karjalainen J, Kujala UM, Stolt A, et al. Angiotensinogen gene M235T polymorphism predicts left ventricular hypertrophy in endurance athletes. J Am Coll Cardiol 1999;34:494–9.
34. Rawlings J, Carre F, Dervio G, et al. Ethnic differences in physiological cardiac adaptations to intense physical exercise in highly trained female athletes. Circulation 2010;121:1078–85.
35. Corrado D, McKenna WJ. Appropriate interpretation of the athlete's electrocardiogram saves lives as well as money. Eur Heart J 2007;28:1920–2.
36. Pelliccia A, Culasso F, Di Paolo F, et al. Prevalence of abnormal electrocardiograms in a large, unselected population undergoing pre-participating cardiovascular screening. Eur Heart J 2007;28:2006–10.
37. Sharma S, Whyte G, Elliott P, et al. Electrocardiographic changes in 1000 highly trained junior elite athletes. Br J Sports Med 1999;33:319–24.
38. Foote CB, Michaud GF. The athlete's electrocardiogram distinguishing normal from abnormal. In: Estes NA, Salem DN, Wang PJ, editors. Sudden cardiac death in the athlete. Armonk (NY): Futura Publishing; 1998. p. 101–3.
39. Wu J, Stork TL, Perron AD, et al. The athlete's electrocardiogram. Am J Emerg Med 2006;24:77–86.
40. Holly RG, Shaffrath JD, Amsterdam EA. Electrocardiographic alterations associated with the hearts of athletes. Sports Med 1998;25:139–48.

41. Maron BJ, Seidman JG, Seidman CE. Proposal for contemporary screening strategies in families with hypertrophic cardiomyopathy. J Am Coll Cardiol 2004;44: 2125–32.
42. Marcus FI, McKenna WJ, Sherrill D, et al. Diagnosis of arrhythmogenic right ventricular cardiomyopathy/dysplasia: proposed modification of the task force criteria. Circulation 2010;121:1533–41.
43. Corrado D, Michieli P, Schiavon M, et al. Prevalence and clinical significance of right precordial T-wave inversion at electrocardiographic preparticipation screening: a prospective study on 3086 young competitive athletes. Circulation 2007;116:339 [abstract: 3392].
44. Papadakis M, Basavarajaiah S, Rawlins J, et al. Prevalence and significance of T-wave inversions in predominantly Caucasian adolescent athletes. Eur Heart J 2009;30(14):1728–35.
45. Myerburg RJ, Vetter VL. Electrocardiograms should be included in pre-participation screening of athletes. Circulation 2007;116:2616–26.
46. Maron BJ. National electrocardiography screening for competitive athletes: feasible in the United States. Ann Intern Med 2010;152:24–6.
47. Chaitman BR. An electrocardiogram should not be included in routine pre-participation screening of young athletes. Circulation 2007;116:2610–4.
48. Corrado D, Basso C, Schiavon M, et al. Screening for hypertrophic cardiomyopathy in young athletes. N Engl J Med 1998;339:364–9.
49. Corrado D, Pelliccia A, Bjornstad HH, et al. Cardiovascular pre-participation screening of young competitive athletes for prevention of sudden death: proposal for a common European protocol. Consensus Statement of the Study Group of Sport Cardiology of the Working Group of Cardiac Rehabilitation and Exercise Physiology and the Working Group of Myocardial and Pericardial Diseases of the European Society of Cardiology. Eur Heart J 2005;26:516–24.
50. Corrado D, Basso C, Pavei A, et al. Trends in cardiovascular sudden death in young competitive athletes after implementation of a preparticipation screening program. J Am Med Assoc 2006;296:1593–601.
51. Sedehi D, Ashley EA. Defining the limits of athlete's heart: implication for screening in diverse populations. Circulation 2010;121:1066–8.
52. Pellica A, Maron BJ, Spataro A, et al. The upper limit of physiological cardiac hypertrophy in highly trained elite athletes. N Engl J Med 1991;324:295–301.
53. Maron BJ. Hypertrophic cardiomyopathy: a systematic review. JAMA 2002;287: 1308–20.
54. Maron BJ, Pellica A. The heart of trained athletes: cardiac remodeling and the risk of sports, including sudden death. Circulation 2006;114:1633–44.
55. Harris KM, Spirito P, Maron MS, et al. Prevalence, clinical profile and significance of left ventricular remodeling in the end-stage phase of hypertrophic cardiomyopathy. Circulation 2006;114:216–25.
56. Lewis JA, Spirito P, Pellica A, et al. Usefulness of Doppler echocardiographic assessment of diastolic filling in distinguishing "athlete's heart" from hypertrophic cardiomyopathy. Br Heart J 1992;68:296–300.
57. Vinereanu D, Florescu N, Schulthorpe N, et al. Differentiation between pathologic and physiologic left ventricular hypertrophy by tissue Doppler assessment of long-axis function in patients with hypertrophic cardiomyopathy or systemic hypertension and in athletes. Am J Cardiol 2001;88:53–8.
58. Richers C, Wilke NM, Jerosch-Herold M, et al. Utility of cardiac magnetic resonance imaging in the diagnosis of hypertrophic cardiomyopathy. Circulation 2005;112:855–61.

59. Maron BJ, Haas TS, Lesser JR. Diagnostic utility of cardiac magnetic resonance imaging in monozygotic twins with hypertrophic cardiomyopathy and identical pattern of left ventricular hypertrophy. Circulation 2007;115:e627–8.

60. Maron MS, Maron BJ, Harrigan C, et al. Hypertrophic cardiomyopathy phenotype revisited at 50 years with cardiovascular magnetic resonance. J Am Coll Cardiol 2009;54:220–8.

61. Pellica A, Maron BJ, Culasso F, et al. Athlete's heart in women: echocardiographic characterization of highly trained elite female athletes. JAMA 1996;276:211–5.

62. Maron MS, Appelbaum E, Harrigan C, et al. Clinical profile and significance of delayed enhancement in hypertrophic cardiomyopathy. Circ Heart Fail 2008;1: 184–91.

63. Ho CY, Lopez B, Coelho-Filho OR, et al. Myocardial fibrosis as an early manifestation of hypertrophic cardiomyopathy. N Engl J Med 2010;363:552–63.

64. Pelliccia A, Spataro A, Maron BJ. Prospective echocardiographic screening for coronary artery anomalies in 1,360 elite competitive athletes. Am J Cardiol 1993;72:978–9.

65. Perloff JK. Congenital heart disease in adults: a new cardiovascular subspecialty. Circulation 1991;84:1881–90.

66. Hutter AM. Cardiovascular abnormalities in the athlete: role of the physician. J Am Coll Cardiol 1994;24:851–3.

67. Maron BJ, Brown RW, McGrew CA, et al. Ethical, legal, and practical considerations affecting medical decision making in competitive athletes. J Am Coll Cardiol 1994;24:854–61.

68. Wyman RA, Chiury RY, Rahko PS. The 5-minute screening echocardiogram. J Am Soc Echocardiogr 2008;21:786–9.

Pulmonary Disorders in Athletes

Max M. Weder, MD*, Jonathon D. Truwit, MD, MBA

KEYWORDS

- Athletes • Exercise • Exercise-induced bronchospasm
- Vocal cord dysfunction

Exercise is rarely limited by pulmonary causes in normal individuals. Cardiac output and peripheral muscle disease are usually the limiting factors. Although minute ventilation rises steeply during exercise, normal individuals maintain a substantial breathing reserve. Exercise in patients, however, can be limited by pulmonary disorders. Acute pulmonary causes (exercise-induced bronchospasm [EIB], vocal cord dysfunction [VCD], exercise-induced anaphylaxis, and exercise-induced urticaria) or chronic disorders (obstructive and restrictive lung disorders) reduce exercise tolerance. Exercise testing has proved the mainstay for diagnosis and treatment of these disorders.

ACUTE PULMONARY DISORDERS AND EXERCISE

Exercise in normal subjects is not limited by the respiratory system. Acute pulmonary disorders are not uncommon in competitive athletes or in athletic individuals. EIB and VCD are the two most common and disabling acute pulmonary disorders in competitive athletes.

Exercise-Induced Bronchospasm

EIB or asthma refers to airway obstruction that occurs in association with exercise in patients with or without a prior history of asthma. Frequently, EIB develops after the exercise period has already ceased. EIB has been reported to occur in up to 80% to 90% of individuals with known asthma[1] and in 10% of the general population without any asthma history.[1] Some believe that all asthmatics will develop EIB given a sufficient exercise load.

Competitive athletes seem to have a high prevalence of asthma and EIB, in particular those athletes participating in winter endurance sports.[2–9] Active asthma in summer athletes was highest in those competing in cycling and mountain biking events (45%) whereas the lowest prevalence was seen in weight lifters and divers (0%).[8] The prevalence of active asthma in those athletes competing in water sports

The authors have nothing to disclose.
Division of Pulmonary and Critical Care Medicine, University of Virginia Health System, PO Box 800546, Charlottesville, VA 22903-0546, USA
* Corresponding author.
E-mail address: Mmw4d@virginia.edu

ranged between 13.8% and 25.9%. Track and field athletes had a prevalence of 12.6% yet gymnasts and fencers had a rate of 2.8%.

Symptoms of EIB may include wheezing, cough, and shortness of breath or chest pain. Wheezing is commonly absent and postexercise cough may be the only symptom, however.[10,11] Of particular concern is that a considerable portion of athletes with objectively documented EIB may not report any symptoms of bronchospasm.[12]

Generally it takes 5 to 8 minutes of strenuous exercise to invoke EIB, and symptoms peak 5 to 10 minutes after cessation of exercise before dissipating at 30 minutes.[13]

Pathogenesis

Despite advancements that led to a better understanding of the pathomechanisms involved in the development of EIB, the exact pathogenesis is incompletely understood. Currently, one of the most widely accepted theories for EIB is an increase in airway osmolarity due to exercise-induced hyperventilation.[14] Vigorous exercise normally results in inhalation of large volumes of cold and dry air, and the subsequent heat loss from the respiratory mucosa induces osmolarity changes, which may, in turn, cause release of proinflammatory cytokines, such as histamine, leukotrienes, and chemokines, by activated epithelial and mast cells.[15] Although it is becoming increasingly clear that alterations in the immune response are pathogenically important in EIB, there seems considerable heterogeneity in the cytokines that are involved in this process. The degree of EIB has been correlated with endothelin-1,[16] phospholipase A2,[17] eosinophils,[18] eosinophilic cationic protein,[19] and lipoxin A4.[20]

Diagnosis

In addition to a compatible history suggesting symptoms of EIB, diagnosis needs to be confirmed by means of objective diagnostic testing. Generally, a fall in forced expiratory volume in the first second of expiration (FEV_1) of 10% or more after an appropriate challenge test is an accepted threshold to diagnose EIB.[21] There is currently no accepted gold standard for diagnosis of EIB. Self-reported symptoms alone that are suggestive of EIB, such as shortness of breath, wheezing, cough, and chest pain, in association with exercise are insufficient to diagnose EIB. Although self-reported symptoms seem specific for EIB, sensitivity is highly variable.[22,23]

EIB can also be diagnosed by methacholine or histamine challenge testing.[24] Methacholine is preferred over histamine because it has fewer systemic side effects. A positive metacholine challenge, however, does not imply the presence of inflammatory cells or mediators known to be present in EIB.[25] Therefore, it is not surprising that the reported sensitivities and specificities for metacholine testing in the diagnosis of EIB are variable. Metacholine testing should not be relied on for diagnosing EIB, and a negative metacholine challenge is insufficient to reliably exclude EIB.[21]

Eucapnic voluntary hyperpnea in the diagnosis of EIB is based on the assumption that increased minute ventilation during exercise is causing airway constriction in susceptible individuals. This diagnostic modality requires subjects to increase minute ventilation to 80% to 85% of the predicted maximum minute ventilation for 5 to 6 minutes, which resembles conditions during vigorous exercise and is used as a substitute. Eucapnic voluntary hyperpnea is the challenge recommended by the International Olympic Committee to diagnose EIB in Olympic athletes.[26] Nonetheless, there is considerable variability in reported sensitivity and specificity, with a high percentage of false-positive test results in some studies. Therefore, it cannot be concluded that this diagnostic tool can substitute for a regular exercise challenge. It is unclear at this point if eucapnic voluntary hyperpnea offers some additional diagnostic value in subjects with inconclusive results on exercise challenge testing.[27]

Mannitol provocation is a technique that has been developed more recently as a tool to diagnose EIB. It simulates an increase in airway osmolarity and initiation of an inflammatory cascade that develops in susceptible individuals during EIB. This challenge can be performed with limited equipment resources and does not require a subject to exercise. Mannitol can be administered via metered dose inhaler, and lung function can subsequently be assessed with simple spirometry. A fall in FEV_1 by 15% or more with mannitol doses of less than 635 mg or a 10% drop with administration of subsequent doses is considered positive.[28] Although the simplicity of mannitol challenge testing is intriguing, its validity in the diagnosis of EIB needs to be confirmed in larger cohorts.

Exercise challenge testing on a treadmill or ergometer according to published American Thoracic Society guidelines[29] is the most widely accepted method of diagnosing EIB. Although a cycle ergometer is more suited for sophisticated measurements, the treadmill may be more likely to induce bronchospasm due to increased minute ventilations for the same level of workload. Well-designed computer programs are now in use to control the test and apply workloads in a standard fashion. The objective is to achieve 6 minutes of exercise at 80% to 85% predicted heart rate maximum in a dry air-conditioned environment.[29] Serial spirometry measurements are then taken after exercise cessation and a 15% drop in FEV_1 is diagnostic for EIB. Care should be taken to assure that short-acting bronchodilators have been withheld for 12 hours and long-acting bronchodilators for 24 hours. Caution in performing the test should be exercised when the pretest FEV_1 is below 70% or 80% of a subject's personal best.[29]

Preventive therapy

Prevention of EIB requires successful treatment of chronic asthma if present, because effective therapy for EIB is unlikely to succeed if airway obstruction is present before exercise. Nonpharmacologic options include induction of a relative refractory period before the exercise event, controlling the climatic conditions. This is generally performed 45 to 60 minutes before the exercise event. Sufficient pre-event exercise loading is required so as to provoke EIB. The degree of refractoriness seems correlated with the extent of bronchospasm induced by the pre-event exercise. Cool and dry air have an impact on the extent of bronchospasm associated with EIB and should be avoided when possible. Nasal breathing or use of a surgical mask or scarf reduces water loss and warms inspired air. Avoidance of winter sports and choosing to exercise indoors under climate-controlled conditions minimizes the occurrence of EIB as well. High dietary salt intake has been suggested to contribute to EIB, and a rise in dietary sodium intake is also a potential factor responsible for the increasing prevalence of asthma in Western industrialized countries. There are some encouraging data suggesting that dietary salt restriction may improve symptomatic control of EIB. The evidence is clinically not convincing enough, however, to suggest that this intervention can substitute for conventional pharmacotherapy. Instead, this should be seen as a potential adjunct.[30–34]

Dietary supplements that have some anti-inflammatory properties, such as fish oil and ascorbic acid, may also provide some benefit in controlling symptoms of EIB, although this evidence is derived from small case series and has not been confirmed in larger clinical trials.[18–21]

Pharmacologic therapy

Primary pharmacologic options include short-acting β-agonists (SABAs), long-acting β-agonists (LABAs), anticholinergics, mast cell stabilizers, leuktotriene receptor antagonists, and inhaled corticosteroids.

SABAs have been the mainstay of therapy for EIB for many years. Inhaled β_2-adrenergic agents are effective in ameliorating or attenuating EIB in 90% of patients. Furthermore, SABAs are the agents of choice as rescue medicines should EIB develop. Unfortunately, tachyphylaxis likely develops in individuals who are using SABAs on a regular basis and this limitation in effectiveness is seen to a lesser degree in the more recently available LABAs as well. Although available evidence indicates that both SABAs and LABAs are effective in preventing EIB, both classes of drugs have been shown less effective in the prevention of EIB when they are used on a daily basis rather than on an as-needed basis.

Two large trials in asthmatic patients have shown that monotherapy with LABAs may increase the risk of exacerbations and treatment failures in subjects previously treated with inhaled corticosteroids.[35] Another trial demonstrated a slight increase in asthma-related and respiratory-related deaths and life-threatening events in asthma patients receiving the LABA salmeterol as monotherapy.[36] Although it is unclear if these data can be applied to subjects with EIB, the use of LABAs as monotherapy in patients with asthma should be discouraged. Similarly, LABAs in combination with inhaled corticosteroids should only be used in asthmatics when symptomatic control cannot be achieved with inhaled corticosteroids alone.

Mast cell stabilizers are not as effective in preventing EIB when compared with β_2-adrenergic agents[37] but more effective than short-acting anticholinergics.[37] Nedocromil sodium and sodium cromoglycate have similar efficacy in prevention of EIB.[38] Up to 40% of patients do not develop EIB after inhaling cromolyn sodium, and approximately 75% derive some degree of protection.[39] Compared with placebo, mast cell stabilizers improve postexercise FEV_1 by an average of approximately 50%.[27] Optimal dosing of cromolyn is 1600 μg 4 times daily with an additional dose 15 minutes before exercise.

Eucosanoids are precursors of cytokines, such as leukotrienes and thromboxane, that can lead to direct bronchoconstriction and result in an inflammatory state that can worsen asthma symptoms. The eucosanoid pathway can be inhibited at different levels by blocking leukotriene receptors (montelukast and zafirlukast), which inhibit lipoxygenase, blocking the enzyme needed to convert arachidonic acid to leukotrienes (zileuton), and by blocking the thromboxane receptor (ramatroban and seratrodast). Leukotriene receptor antagonists are a new class of drugs that have proved effective in providing symptomatic control in subjects with mild to moderate asthma. Their effectiveness in the prevention of EIB and low potential for side effects have been demonstrated in several well-designed clinical trials.[40–47] The lipoxygenase inhibitor zileuton offers comparable protection but has a shorter duration of action.[41] Thromboxane inhibitors are not commercially available for asthma therapy. Limited data suggest that ramatroban effectively prevents EIB in subjects with mild pre-existing asthma.[48] Although preclinical data suggest that seratrodast ameliorates the proinflammatory states in subjects with asthma,[49] it has not yet been studied in EIB.

Although there is abundant evidence to support the use of inhaled corticosteroids to control symptoms in patients with asthma,[50] their role in the treatment of EIB is less clear, particularly in those subjects without pre-existing asthma. The data on the use of a single dose of an inhaled corticosteroid to prevent the onset of EIB are conflicting. The pooled results of 4 crossover trials showed no difference between single-dose inhaled corticosteroids and placebo in the prevention of EIB.[27]

Training goals in athletes with EIB are no different than for normal subjects. Clark and Cochrane[51] have outlined a method to help asthmatics define the exercise level needed to achieve 75% heart rate maximum but maintain their dyspnea index (minute ventilation [VE]/maximum voluntary ventilation [MVV]) below 60%. When $\dot{V}_E$/MVV exceeds 60%, it is unlikely that exercise will be maintained for greater than 15 minutes.

Asthmatic athletes may undergo incremental exercise testing to determine the training intensity at which a 70% heart rate maximum with a V_E/MVV ratio less than 60% is achieved. Asthmatics should choose their exercise and training activities carefully, realizing that cold, dry air exacerbates asthma and is a major factor in inducing EIB. Activities that do not generate high minute ventilations (tennis, handball, racquetball, karate, wrestling, boxing, golf, sprinting, isometrics, downhill skiing, football, and baseball) are preferred as are water activities (swimming, diving, and water polo). Activities with high minute ventilation (long distance running, cycling, basketball, soccer, and rugby) or those taking place in a cool and dry climate (ice hockey, ice skating, and cross-country skiing) are more likely to induce EIB.[7,8,29,52,53]

Vocal Cord Dysfunction

VCD is a syndrome of inappropriate vocal cord adduction during the respiratory cycle resulting in wheezing and shortness of breath.[54] Patients may complain of inability to get air in. They often point to their upper trachea as the region of concern. Audible upper airway wheezing is appreciated and lack of responsiveness to bronchodilators is the rule. It occurs more frequently in women than in men and commonly presents in individuals between 20 and 40 years of age.[54,55] Between 1984 and 1991, National Jewish Hospital identified 95 patients referred with refractory asthma as having VCD (44% with VCD alone and 56% with VCD and asthma).[54] Patients with VCD alone were more likely to have emergency department visits in the year preceding referral (9.7 vs 5.5).

Diagnosis
On physical examination, rapid breathing is noted at or near residual volume. Inspiratory wheezing is localized to the larynx and is not well transmitted to the thorax but still causes many patients with VCD to be misdiagnosed with asthma.[56] Hyperinflation is generally not appreciated. One-fourth have evidence of truncated inspiratory limb on flow-volume loops, which indicates extrathoracic airway obstruction.[54] Pulmonary function testing is variable and often not reproducible. Furthermore, pulmonary function testing demonstrates no response to β_2-adrenergic agonists. Arterial blood sample analysis is usually normal. Laryngoscopy is the mainstay of diagnosis but is only 60% sensitive during an asymptomatic period. Its sensitivity approaches 100% during an attack of VCD. Laryngoscopy may reveal vocal cord adduction during inspiration or early expiration.[54,57] The adduction is more prominent in the anterior portion of the cords, creating a diamond-shaped passage.

Psychiatric diagnoses are common in patients with vocal cord dysfunction. Of those with psychiatric diagnoses, 73% have an Axis I diagnosis whereas 37% have an Axis II diagnosis.[54,57,58] Physical, sexual, and/or emotional abuses are more common in patients with VCD than in asthmatics.

Because many of these patients are referred for EIB, pulmonary function testing and exercise testing can be useful to distinguish VCD from EIB. Evidence of upper airway obstruction is often elucidated during an exercise test.[58] Laryngoscopy can be performed once signs of VCD are triggered from exercise. Newer exercise test equipment permits real-time flow-loop displays, which allow for detection of the variable extrathoracic upper airway obstruction.

Therapy
Treatment is effective both for immediate relief and prevention. Various breathing maneuvers have been reported to effectively abort an attack of VCD, including rapid shallow breathing (panting)[59]; diaphragmatic breathing, breathing through the nose;

Pulmonary Function Analysis

Spirometry	Predicted (Favor Mean)	Predicted (Favor Range)	Predrug Reported	Predrug (% Predicted)	Postdrug Reported	Postdrug (% Predicted)	Change (%)
FVC	5.52	>4.52	6.41	116	6.58	119	3
FEV$_1$	4.70	>3.88	5.56	118	5.89	125	6
FEV$_1$/FVC	86.96	>77.19	88.67	100	89.48	103	3
FEF$_{25\%-75\%}$	463	>2.84	6.23	134	7.15	154	15
FEF$_{max}$	8.98	>6.49	11 20	125	9.73	109	−13
TET	—	—	6.25	—	7.62	—	22
Lung Volumes	Predicted (Favor Mean)	Predicted (Favor Range)	Predrug Reported	Predrug (% Predicted)	Postdrug Reported	Postdrug (% Predicted)	Change (%)
VC	5.52	>4.52	5.67	103	5.82	105	3
TLC	7.58	7.58	8.48	112	6.94	92	−18
RV	1.43	1.43	2.81	196	1.12	78	−60
RV/TLC	15.39	15.39	33.10	215	18.09	105	−51
FRC	3.15	3.15	3.86	123	2.39	76	−38
ERV	1.87	1.87	1.05	57	1.28	68	21
RAW	0.20–2.50	0.20–2.50	2.27	—	3.15	—	39
SGaw	0.11–0.40	0.11–0.40	0.12	—	0.13	—	10
Diffusion							

	Predicted (Favor Mean)	Predicted (Favor Range)	Predrug Reported	Predrug (% Predicted)	Postdrug Reported	Postdrug (% Predicted)	Change (%)
Dsb	41.56	41.56	40.70	96	—	—	—
DsbHb	41.56	41.56	40.70	98	—	—	—
VAsb	7.33	7.33	7.44	102	—	—	—
D/VAsb	5.63	5.63	5.47	97	—	—	—
D/VAsb	5.63	5.63	5.47	97	—	—	—
Vinsp	—	—	5.93	—	—	—	—

Abbreviations: Dsb, Diffusion, single breath; DsbHb, diffusion, single breath, adjusted for hemoglobin; D/VAsb, Diffusion in relation to single breath alveolar volume; ERV, expiratory reserve volume; FRC, functional residual capacity; RV, residual volume; RAW, airway resistance; SGaw, specific airway conductance; TET, total expiratory time; TLC, total lung capacity; VAsb, alveolar volume, single breath; VC, vital capacity; Vinsp, inspiratory volume.

breathing through a straw, pursed-lip breathing; and breathing with a hissing sound. The administration of an oxygen/helium mixture (heliox) may reduce airway resistance and rapidly improve VCD.[60]

Long-term management of VCD should include treatment or elimination of potential triggers, such as gastroesophageal reflux disease, rhinosinusitis, psychological stressors, and airborne irritants. Speech pathology is considered the mainstay of long-term management for VCD and has effectively alleviated symptoms and prevented recurrence.[56,61] Psychological counseling may be helpful in the appropriate setting. Biofeedback[62] and hypnosis[63] have been used in the treatment of VCD, but this approach is only supported by limited evidence. Anxiolytics may be effective to abort acute episodes of VCD[64] and can be appropriate to alleviate anxiety attacks in the short term, but their long-term use for management of VCD should be discouraged. Buspirone has been effective in patients with VCD (Jonathon Truwit, MD, personal communication, November 1, 2010). Doses as low as 5 mg, 3 times daily, may be sufficient, but on occasion doses of 15 mg, 3 times daily, have been needed.

Limited evidence suggests that pretreatment with short-acting anticholinergic medications may be able to alleviate exercise-induced VCD.[56]

Cough and/or Chest pain

Cough and chest pain are common symptoms in athletic individuals and may be presenting symptoms of EIB. Other diagnoses must be entertained. In young healthy individuals, noncardiac causes dominate but as subjects age, cardiac chest pain becomes more prominent.

Common noncardiac causes include pleuritis, pleurodynia, bronchitis, pneumonia, costochondritis, intercostal muscle strains, and chest wall trauma. Less common considerations should include pneumothorax, pleural effusion, pulmonary embolism, esophageal reflux or spasm, cervical disk disease, arthritis, breast disorders, herpes zoster, panic attacks, and performance anxiety. Cardiac causes include angina, ventricular and supraventricular arrhythmias, pericarditis, Wolff-Parkinson-White syndrome, cocaine usage, hypertrophic cardiomyopathy, mitral valve prolapse, aortic stenosis, and aortic dissection.

Common causes of cough include bronchitis, postnasal drip, sinusitis, pneumonia, postviral bronchospasm, tonsillitis, laryngitis, and EIB. Less common causes include infectious causes (tuberculosis, fungal, and *Pneumocystis carinii* pneumonia), drug induced (angiotensin-converting enzyme inhibitors and β-blockers), gastroesophageal reflux disease, aspiration, foreign body aspiration, tumors (bronchogenic, mediastinal, and laryngeal), interstitial lung diseases, congenital anomalies, local irritants, and posttraumatic.

SUMMARY

The respiratory system rarely limits exercise in normal subjects. In patients with chronic pulmonary processes or in the elite athlete, however, the respiratory system may be a limiting factor. Common respiratory disorders include chest pain syndromes, cough, exercise-induced asthma, and vocal cord dysfunction. Exercise testing can be useful to distinguish acute and chronic pulmonary causes of dyspnea during exercise as well as to differentiate between cardiac and pulmonary causes (Appendix 1).

APPENDIX 1: FROM TEXT TO PRACTICE: CLINICAL APPLICATION OF ARTICLE MATERIAL

An 18-year-old college freshman complains of trouble breathing in association with rowing. She notes no wheezing but does feel chest tightness on deep inspiration.

She has experienced this while rowing competitively in high school. It only occurs during strenuous workouts that simulate races or during an actual race. These workouts consist of 2 intense 10-minute sessions with a few minutes of rest between. The onset of her symptoms is during the second minute of the second session. She feels like her breathing recovers more slowly than that of her teammates. Cold air makes her feel like she has an "icy burn" in her airway. She has no history of postnasal drip or acid reflux. She did try montelukast (Singulair) for 5 to 6 days. She is not sure that it helped, perhaps on the first day or so. Today she feels some chest tightness at rest, especially with a deep breath. Last week she had exercise spirometry. FEV_1; forced vital capacity (FVC); and forced expiratory flow (FEF), midexpiratory phase$_{25\%-75\%}$ were normal at baseline (5.00, 5.68, and 5.48, respectively). Patient exercised 10 minutes at 5.6 to 7.2 mph on 10% to 13% incline. She did not show an appreciable decline in postexercise spirometry.

The table lists her pulmonary function tests.

Diagnosis: asthma.

Despite her normal spirometry and negative exercise spirometry study, the patient's lung volumes reveal air trapping and substantial improvement with bronchodilator therapy. Spirometry is the most practical means of diagnosing asthma. When spirometry is normal but there is a high clinical suspicion for asthma, however, the clinician should pursue additional testing. This may include exercise spirometry, lung volumes, or methacholine challenge test.

REFERENCES

1. McFadden ER Jr, Gilbert IA. Exercise-induced asthma. N Engl J Med 1994;330: 1362.
2. Fitch KD. Management of allergic Olympic athletes. J Allergy Clin Immunol 1984; 73:722.
3. Larsson K, Ohlsen P, Larsson L, et al. High prevalence of asthma in cross country skiers. BMJ 1993;307:1326.
4. Nystad W. Asthma. Int J Sports Med 2000;21(Suppl 2):S98.
5. Rice SG, Bierman CW, Shapiro GG, et al. Identification of exercise-induced asthma among intercollegiate athletes. Ann Allergy 1985;55:790.
6. Voy RO, The US. Olympic Committee experience with exercise-induced bronchospasm. Med Sci Sports Exerc 1984;18(328):1986.
7. Weiler JM, Ryan EJ 3rd. Asthma in United States Olympic athletes who participated in the 1998 Olympic winter games. J Allergy Clin Immunol 2000;106:267.
8. Weiler JM, Layton T, Hunt M. Asthma in United States Olympic athletes who participated in the 1996 Summer Games. J Allergy Clin Immunol 1998;102:722.
9. Weiler JM, Metzger WJ, Donnelly AL, et al. Prevalence of bronchial hyperresponsiveness in highly trained athletes. Chest 1986;90:23.
10. Anderson S. Exercise-induced asthma. In: Middleton E, Reed C, Ellis E, et al, editors. Allergy: principles and practice. 4th edition. St Louis (MO): Mosby; 1993. p. 1343.
11. Lemanske RF Jr, Henke K. Exercise-induced asthma. In: Gisolfi C, Lamb D, editors, Perspectives in exercise and sports medicine: youth, exercise and sport, vol. 2. Indianapolis (IN): Benchmark Press; 1989. p. 465.
12. Parsons JP, Kaeding C, Phillips G, et al. Prevalence of exercise-induced bronchospasm in a cohort of varsity college athletes. Med Sci Sports Exerc 2007;39:1487.
13. Anderson S, Seale JP, Ferris L, et al. An evaluation of pharmacotherapy for exercise-induced asthma. J Allergy Clin Immunol 1979;64:612.

14. Weiler JM, Bonini S, Coifman R, et al. American Academy of Allergy, Asthma & Immunology Work Group report: exercise-induced asthma. J Allergy Clin Immunol 2007;119:1349.
15. McFadden ER Jr, Nelson JA, Skowronski ME, et al. Thermally induced asthma and airway drying. Am J Respir Crit Care Med 1999;160:221.
16. Zietkowski Z, Skiepko R, Tomasiak MM, et al. Endothelin-1 in exhaled breath condensate of allergic asthma patients with exercise-induced bronchoconstriction. Respir Res 2007;8:76.
17. Hallstrand TS, Chi EY, Singer AG, et al. Secreted phospholipase A2 group X overexpression in asthma and bronchial hyperresponsiveness. Am J Respir Crit Care Med 2007;176:1072.
18. Duong M, Subbarao P, Adelroth E, et al. Sputum eosinophils and the response of exercise-induced bronchoconstriction to corticosteroid in asthma. Chest 2008; 133:404.
19. Hsieh CC, Goto H, Kobayashi H, et al. Changes in serum eosinophil cationic protein levels after exercise challenge in asthmatic children. J Asthma 2007;44:569.
20. Tahan F, Saraymen R, Gumus H. The role of lipoxin A4 in exercise-induced bronchoconstriction in asthma. J Asthma 2008;45:161.
21. Crapo RO, Casaburi R, Coates AL, et al. Guidelines for methacholine and exercise challenge testing-1999. This official statement of the American Thoracic Society was adopted by the ATS Board of Directors, July 1999. Am J Respir Crit Care Med 2000;161:309.
22. Kyle JM, Walker RB, Hanshaw SL, et al. Exercise-induced bronchospasm in the young athlete: guidelines for routine screening and initial management. Med Sci Sports Exerc 1992;24:856.
23. Rupp NT, Brudno DS, Guill MF. The value of screening for risk of exercise-induced asthma in high school athletes. Ann Allergy 1993;70:339.
24. AARC clinical practice guideline. Bronchial provocation. American Association for Respiratory Care. Respir Care 1992;37:902.
25. Anderson SD, Holzer K. Exercise-induced asthma: is it the right diagnosis in elite athletes? J Allergy Clin Immunol 2000;106:419.
26. Rundell KW, Slee JB. Exercise and other indirect challenges to demonstrate asthma or exercise-induced bronchoconstriction in athletes. J Allergy Clin Immunol 2008;122:238.
27. Dryden DM, Spooner CH, Stickland MK, et al. Exercise-induced bronchoconstriction and asthma. Evid Rep Technol Assess (Full Rep) 2010;189:1–154, v–vi.
28. Holzer K, Anderson SD, Chan HK, et al. Mannitol as a challenge test to identify exercise-induced Bronchoconstriction in elite athletes. Am J Resp Crit Care Med 2003;157:534-7.
29. Crapo RO, Casaburi R, Coates AL, et al. Guidelines for methacholine and exercise challenge testing-1999. This official statement of the American Thoracic Society was adopted by the ATS Board of Directors, July 1999. Am J Respir Crit Care Med 2000;161:309.
30. Mickleborough TD. Salt intake, asthma, and exercise-induced bronchoconstriction: a review. Phys Sportsmed 2010;38:118.
31. Mickleborough TD, Gotshall RW. Dietary salt intake as a potential modifier of airway responsiveness in bronchial asthma. J Altern Complement Med 2004; 10:633.
32. Gotshall RW, Mickleborough TD, Cordain L. Dietary salt restriction improves pulmonary function in exercise-induced asthma. Med Sci Sports Exerc 1815; 32:2000.

33. Mickleborough TD, Lindley MR, Ray S. Dietary salt, airway inflammation, and diffusion capacity in exercise-induced asthma. Med Sci Sports Exerc 2005;37:904.
34. Lazarus SC, Boushey HA, Fahy JV, et al. Long-acting beta2-agonist monotherapy vs continued therapy with inhaled corticosteroids in patients with persistent asthma: a randomized controlled trial. JAMA 2001;285:2583.
35. Lemanske RF Jr, Sorkness CA, Mauger EA, et al. Inhaled corticosteroid reduction and elimination in patients with persistent asthma receiving salmeterol: a randomized controlled trial. JAMA 2001;285:2594.
36. Nelson HS, Weiss ST, Bleecker ER, et al. The Salmeterol Multicenter Asthma Research Trial: a comparison of usual pharmacotherapy for asthma or usual pharmacotherapy plus salmeterol. Chest 2006;129:15.
37. Spooner CH, Spooner GR, Rowe BH. Mast-cell stabilising agents to prevent exercise-induced bronchoconstriction. Cochrane Database Syst Rev 2003;4: CD002307.
38. Kelly K, Spooner CH, Rowe BH. Nedocromil sodium vs. sodium cromoglycate for preventing exercise-induced bronchoconstriction in asthmatics. Cochrane Database Syst Rev 2000;4:CD002731.
39. Godfrey S, Konig P. Inhibition of exercise-induced asthma by different pharmacological pathways. Thorax 1976;31:137.
40. Rundell KW, Spiering BA, Baumann JM, et al. Effects of montelukast on airway narrowing from eucapnic voluntary hyperventilation and cold air exercise. Br J Sports Med 2005;39:232.
41. Coreno A, Skowronski M, Kotaru C, et al. Comparative effects of long-acting beta2-agonists, leukotriene receptor antagonists, and a 5-lipoxygenase inhibitor on exercise-induced asthma. J Allergy Clin Immunol 2000;106:500.
42. Mastalerz L, Gawlewicz-Mroczka A, Nizankowska E, et al. Protection against exercise-induced bronchoconstriction by montelukast in aspirin-sensitive and aspirin-tolerant patients with asthma. Clin Exp Allergy 2002;32:1360.
43. Pearlman DS, Ostrom NK, Bronsky EA, et al. The leukotriene D4-receptor antagonist zafirlukast attenuates exercise-induced bronchoconstriction in children. J Pediatr 1999;134:273.
44. Pearlman DS, van Adelsberg J, Philip G, et al. Onset and duration of protection against exercise-induced bronchoconstriction by a single oral dose of montelukast. Ann Allergy Asthma Immunol 2006;97:98.
45. Peroni DG, Piacentini GL, Ress M, et al. Time efficacy of a single dose of montelukast on exercise-induced asthma in children. Pediatr Allergy Immunol 2002;13:434.
46. Philip G, Pearlman DS, Villaran C, et al. Single-dose montelukast or salmeterol as protection against exercise-induced bronchoconstriction. Chest 2007;132:875.
47. Philip G, Villaran C, Pearlman DS, et al. Protection against exercise-induced bronchoconstriction two hours after a single oral dose of montelukast. J Asthma 2007; 44:213.
48. Magnussen H, Boerger S, Templin K, et al. Effects of a thromboxane-receptor antagonist, BAY u 3405, on prostaglandin D2- and exercise-induced bronchoconstriction. J Allergy Clin Immunol 1992;89:1119.
49. Fukuoka T, Miyake S, Umino T, et al. The effect of seratrodast on eosinophil cationic protein and symptoms in asthmatics. J Asthma 2003;40:257.
50. Adams NP, Jones PW. The dose-response characteristics of inhaled corticosteroids when used to treat asthma: an overview of Cochrane systematic reviews. Respir Med 2006;100:1297.
51. Clark CJ, Cochrane LM. Assessment of work performance in asthma for determination of cardiorespiratory fitness and training capacity. Thorax 1988;43:745.

52. Helenius I, Haahtela T. Allergy and asthma in elite summer sport athletes. J Allergy Clin Immunol 2000;106:444.
53. Helenius IJ, Tikkanen HO, Haahtela T. Association between type of training and risk of asthma in elite athletes. Thorax 1997;52:157.
54. Newman KB, Mason UG 3rd, Schmaling KB. Clinical features of vocal cord dysfunction. Am J Respir Crit Care Med 1995;152:1382.
55. Morris MJ, Deal LE, Bean DR, et al. Vocal cord dysfunction in patients with exertional dyspnea. Chest 1999;116:1676.
56. Doshi DR, Weinberger MM. Long-term outcome of vocal cord dysfunction. Ann Allergy Asthma Immunol 2006;96:794.
57. O'Hollaren MT. Masqueraders in clinical allergy: laryngeal dysfunction causing dyspnea. Ann Allergy 1990;65:351.
58. Christopher KL, Wood RP 2nd, Eckert RC, et al. Vocal-cord dysfunction presenting as asthma. N Engl J Med 1983;308:1566.
59. Pitchenik AE. Functional laryngeal obstruction relieved by panting. Chest 1991; 100:1465.
60. Berkenbosch JW, Grueber RE, Graff GR, et al. Patterns of helium-oxygen (heliox) usage in the critical care environment. J Intensive Care Med 2004;19:335.
61. Pargeter N, Mansur A. The effectiveness of speech and language therapy in vocal cord dysfunction. Thorax 2006;61(Suppl 2):ii26.
62. McFadden ER Jr, Zawadski DK. Vocal cord dysfunction masquerading as exercise-induced asthma. a physiologic cause for "choking" during athletic activities. Am J Respir Crit Care Med 1996;153:942.
63. Anbar RD, Hehir DA. Hypnosis as a diagnostic modality for vocal cord dysfunction. Pediatrics 2000;106:E81.
64. Roberts KW, Crnkovic A, Steiniger JR. Post-anesthesia paradoxical vocal cord motion successfully treated with midazolam. Anesthesiology 1998;89:517.

Sickle Cell Considerations in Athletes

E. Randy Eichner, MD*

KEYWORDS

- Sickle cell trait • Sudden death • Rhabdomyolysis
- Splenic infarction • Hematuria

The most vital sickle cell considerations in athletes relate to sickle cell trait (SCT). How SCT can affect athletes is replete with recent advances, updates, and controversies. The key clinical concerns for athletes with SCT are listed in **Box 1**.

These concerns are discussed in this article, along with other clinical concerns for athletes with sickling hemoglobinopathies such as hemoglobin SC, S-beta-thalassemia, and hemoglobin SE disease. Although some children and adolescents with sickle cell anemia (hemoglobin SS) compete in recreational and even team sports, secondary to anemia and cumulative complications from disease, very few compete in varsity sports in high school.[1] Therefore, sickle cell anemia is not addressed in this article.

DEFINITION, FREQUENCY, AND VARIATION OF SICKLE CELL TRAIT

SCT is not a disease but a condition, resulting from inheritance of one gene for sickle hemoglobin (S) and one gene for normal hemoglobin (A). The sickle gene is common in regions endemic with malaria, because SCT protects against early death from malaria, providing a procreation advantage to SCT carriers. SCT is found in about 8% of African American, 0.5% of Hispanic, and 0.2% of white individuals.[2] Each red blood cell in SCT typically has about 40% hemoglobin S. The co-inheritance of alpha-thalassemia trait, which occurs in about one-third of blacks (about 30% have a 1-gene and 2% have a 2-gene deletion of the 4 alpha-globin genes), lowers the amount of hemoglobin S in each red blood cell and may lessen the risk of exertional sickling.[3]

EXERTIONAL SICKLING IN ATHLETES

The most vital clinical consideration for athletes with SCT is exertional sickling, because this "sudden-collapse" syndrome can be fatal. Despite increasing national

Disclosure: No funding received for this work. This author has nothing to disclose.
OU Sooner Football, University of Oklahoma Health Sciences Center, Oklahoma City, OK, USA
* 321 Baudin Way, Sonoma, CA 95476-5669.
E-mail address: reichner1@comcast.net

Clin Sports Med 30 (2011) 537–549
doi:10.1016/j.csm.2011.03.004
0278-5919/11/$ – see front matter © 2011 Elsevier Inc. All rights reserved.

Box 1
Clinical concerns among athletes with SCT

1. Exertional sickling collapse
2. Lumbar paraspinal myonecrosis and other compartment syndromes
3. Splenic infarction at altitude
4. Gross hematuria
5. Hyposthenuria
6. Venous thromboembolism (questionable)

---

focus on this problem, fatal cases continue to occur, as illustrated by the demise of a 20-year-old male student-athlete in August 2010 during a track tryout at a university in North Carolina.[4] Other sickling collapses and deaths have occurred in various sports or exercises (**Box 2**), and have included male and female athletes, some as young as 12 years old.[5–7] Litigation over exertional sickling deaths of college football players has led to decisions by the National Collegiate Athletic Association (NCAA) on screening for SCT in college athletes. To date, the debate continues on the wisdom of this mandatory screening program and on how best to prevent tragic exertional sickling deaths.[2]

Deaths from exertional sickling have been more common in football players. The first reported case was the death of a fullback in 1963 during preseason training at a university in New Mexico. Few details are available on his death.[8] The first exertional sickling death in college football reported with some description and clinical information was in 1974.[9] A 19-year-old African American with SCT, who was a defensive back and punt returner from Florida, collapsed 2 years in a row on the first day of practice at an altitude of 5400 ft in Colorado. He survived the first year. During the second year, while aiming to finish the first conditioning sprint (880 yards), he fell behind his group at 660 yards, staggered forward, and fell at the edge of the track. He complained of severe leg pain and died the following day while hospitalized with "severe acidosis" and "severe sickling in the kidneys." In addition to these early deaths, at least 20 other deaths have occurred secondary to exertional sickling in college football players. Similar deaths have also occurred in high school and youth league football.[10]

Exertional sickling has become the leading "killer" in NCAA Division-1 football and a recent spate of deaths from exertional sickling in NCAA Division-1 football is illustrative and alarming. An examination of all deaths in Division-1 football during the past decade (2000–2010) revealed zero deaths from "play" of the game, zero deaths from "practice" of the game, and 16 deaths from *conditioning* for the game, including 15

Box 2
Sports settings for exertional sickling collapse

1. Football conditioning
2. Basketball training
3. Cross-country racing
4. University track tryout
5. Golden Gloves boxing bout
6. Recreational ocean swimming

---

from sprinting or high-speed agility drills and 1 from weight lifting. Of these 16 deaths, 4 were cardiac induced, 1 secondary to complications from asthma, and 1 from exertional heat stroke (EHS). An alarming 10 (63%) of these deaths were attributed to complications of exertional sickling. Thus, SCT, carried by an estimated 3% to 4% of all Division-1 football players, accounts for 63% of the deaths, an excess of 16-fold to 21-fold.[6] Before further examining the deaths of college football players and other athletes from exertional sickling, it is relevant to review the experience and research on comparable deaths in military recruits undergoing basic training, which is akin to an "athletics" setting.

Sickling Deaths in Military Recruits

The first report of SCT and sudden death in military recruits was in 1970. During one year of Army basic combat training in El Paso, 4 (0.1%) of 4000 African American recruits died suddenly. All 4 had SCT. One apparently died of coronary heart disease, but the other 3 fit a pattern: collapse during running, hypotension, metabolic acidosis, hyperkalemia, disseminated intravascular coagulation (DIC), oliguria, and "sudden" death 8 to 25 hours after the collapse.[11] As an esteemed sickle-cell expert said, "The four deaths involved only soldiers with SCT; death did not occur in the thousands of soldiers who did not possess the trait…death occurred in more than 1% of those with SCT. It is obvious that SCT was a factor in causing death."[12(p360)]

The pattern was clarified by the next report. From 1970 to 1974, at 2 large military installations, 2 recruits and 2 cadets were hospitalized for exertional rhabdomyolysis, DIC, and renal failure. Three collapsed after a run, and 1 had severe muscle cramping and swelling after a run. All needed early renal dialysis; 1 died of hyperkalemia. All 4 had SCT.[13]

Subsequently, there was a study of all deaths among 2 million recruits during basic training in the US Armed Forces from 1977 through 1981. The risk of unexplained sudden death in black recruits with SCT was 40 times higher than in all other recruits.[14] A follow-up analysis concluded that exercise-related death in black recruits with SCT was 30 times more common than in black recruits without SCT, and that exertional heat illness (EHI) was often the initiating homeostatic dysfunction.[3]

Following this report, a 10-year study (1982–1991) tested the hypothesis that better prevention of EHI would reduce excess SCT deaths. Army drill instructors monitored ambient heat, decreased exercise intensity, and increased rest cycles and hydration with worsening hot weather, and responded early to any individuals who were "struggling." Although this study has been presented and discussed but not published, the intervention seemed to eliminate mortality for recruits with SCT.[15] Therefore, the Army stopped screening recruits for SCT in 1996, stating that preventing EHI prevented most SCT-related deaths, and as a result, screening was not cost-effective.[16]

Despite this prevention program, exercise-related deaths continued in Army recruits with SCT. For example, 6 deaths occurred from 1992 to 2001.[16] Also, a 1967 report of "nephropathy associated with heat stress and exercise" provided a clue that classical EHI was different from the collapse syndrome in recruits with SCT. Seven of 8 cases reported were classical EHI (heatstroke). These 7 were recruits training in the heat of the South and all 7 examined during the acute phase of their illness had rectal temperatures of 104°F to 108°F. But the eighth case was different. He was training in the North and his rectal temperature was only 101°F. From the commencement of training, he had trouble "in completing running." On day 15, he collapsed after running 2 miles. The only black of the 8 recruits, he had SCT. Anuric for 10 days, he survived after dialysis and may be the first reported military case of exertional sickling collapse.[17]

It seems that EHI has been overrated as a trigger for sickling in SCT. In one analysis, Army researchers outlined 30 exercise collapses (21 fatal) in SCT, and concluded that 22 had EHI. Yet, most had core temperatures of 102°F or lower, or had no temperature recorded.[3] Hence, it seems that most had merely the expected physiologic hyperthermia of strenuous exercise that induced collapse.

Analysis of deaths in recruits with SCT also shows that most collapse when running 1 to 3 miles and that many deaths are from metabolic complications of fulminant rhabdomyolysis, including acute renal failure.[3] Even the early deaths within 30 to 60 minutes, often from cardiac arrhythmias including pulseless electrical activity and asystole, are likely caused by complications from fulminant rhabdomyolysis, including hyperkalemia, lactic acidosis, and hypocalcemia.

Accordingly, the main cause of death in exertional sickling is "explosive" rhabdomyolysis, from ischemia. In fact, the risk of fatal rhabdomyolysis in Army recruits with SCT was increased roughly 200-fold[18]; and it seems that, more often than not, the trigger for sickling is not an EHI, but a sudden bout of sustained maximal exertion. Granted, ambient heat can make any drill harder; however, the common trigger is physical intensity. A close look at the college football deaths shows that the pivotal problem is exercise *intensity*.

Problem is Exercise Intensity

Sickling collapses occur "all year round" in football. The typical exercise stimulus for a sickling collapse is maximal exertion sustained for at least a few minutes. It can occur either at the end of an hour-long, fast-tempo station drill, or can occur early, after the athlete has been on-field for only a brief time, sprinting all-out for only 2 to 5 minutes.[6] Some college football collapses have occurred after sprinting a total distance of only 600 to 1200 m. Other problematic situations can include an abrupt increase in intensity of training especially on the first day of physical conditioning, training at unfamiliar altitude, or suboptimal physical conditioning, as is the case in athletes who have recently returned from a vacation. These factors all seem to spawn a "perfect storm" of undue exercise intensity, sustained for at least a few minutes, and a "heroic effort" beyond the physical limits of an athlete with SCT on any given day.[5,6] A few examples illustrate the susceptibility to sickle secondary to high-intensity exercise.

Of the 10 Division-1 football players who died from exertional sickling in the past decade, 5 had been performing serial sprints for 5 to 30 minutes and 4 had been performing fast-tempo, multistation drills, with little or no rest between stations, for 12 to 60 minutes. In 5 earlier deaths of football players with SCT, the sprinting activity that had induced sickling collapse was performed for only 2 to 5 minutes. Of these 5 players, 2 were unaccustomed to training at altitude. And last, a 19-year-old African American college football player in Texas collapsed after a conditioning run on a "mild" day in September. He ran 16 successive sprints of 100 yards each, lagged behind teammates on the final sprints, and on finishing the workout, complained of shortness of breath and leg pain. He was initially alert, yet within 10 minutes became lethargic. Too weak to stand, he was transported to the athletic training room, where despite supportive therapy and intravenous fluids, he lost consciousness within 15 minutes. He was rushed to a hospital, where he was noted to have profound lactic acidosis and fulminant rhabdomyolysis. He developed acute renal failure and DIC, remained unresponsive, and died about 15 hours after collapse—from hyperkalemia and pulseless electrical activity that led to asystole.[19]

In consequence, it appears that the early onset and greater degree of sickling is directly proportional to the intensity of physical activity in athletes with SCT, and is a plausible explanation for earlier sickling collapse in "sprinting" football players compared with "running" military recruits.

Chronology of Pathophysiology and Sickling Collapse

The onset of pathophysiological changes parallels the "timing" of sickling collapses. Sprinting football players can collapse from sickling within 2 to 5 minutes. Maximal exertion can induce profound metabolic changes within 2 to 5 minutes, which can foster sickling collapse in athletes with SCT. For example, physiologic studies in non-SCT subjects show that maximal cycling or running can evoke severe hypoxemia and lactic acidosis within 1 to 5 minutes,[20–22] and that dehydration can increase exertional sickling.[23] Other perturbations that also can develop rapidly, include muscle hyperthermia and dehydration of individual red cells, as they course through the hyperosmotic (high lactate) milieu of working muscles. These 4 adverse forces in concert—profound hypoxemia, lactic acidosis, hyperosmolarity, and red-cell dehydration (which concentrates hemoglobin S)—promote sickling in the microcirculation.[6] Also, in a study of young men with SCT who performed 2, brief, maximal arm-cranking exercise bouts, one bout at 1270 m and the other at a simulated 4000 m, sickle cells (more frequent at altitude) were observed in venous blood from the arm within 2 to 5 minutes.[24]

Intriguing new research

Simply stated, sickle cells are "stiff and sticky" and thus have a propensity to "logjam" small blood vessels and deplete blood supply to working muscles. Several recent studies suggest that SCT carriers, compared with controls, may have impaired blood rheology in the microcirculation secondary to amplified red cell rigidity, blood viscosity, and endothelial adhesion.[25–27] However, the effects of diverse, laboratory-based exercise bouts on these parameters have been moderate and varied. Hydration, as compared with a dehydrated milieu, can improve blood viscosity and, in turn, enhance blood rheology during exercise, which has practical implications for athletes with SCT.[28]

Recent muscle biopsy research shows remodeling of microvasculature in SCT carriers, with reduced numbers of narrow capillaries, yet increased numbers of wide capillaries, perhaps reflective of an adaptation to promote blood flow in the presence of rigid red cells and elevated blood viscosity.[29] Most laboratory-based studies show that exercise performance in individuals with SCT is the same as controls, including brief, supramaximal exercise.[30] In contrast, one study showed a different pattern of repeated sprint ability in individuals with SCT. During five, 6-second bouts of maximal cycling sprints, interspersed with 24 seconds of rest, the total work done was the same, yet peak power output declined faster in SCT carriers compared with controls.[31] Whether this reflects impaired rheology from exertional sickling is unknown. And, another recent study with practical implications, suggests that habitual physical activity may decrease endothelial activation in SCT, which may limit the risk for exertional sickling events.[32]

Differentiating Sickling Collapse

Not all sickling collapses are identical, but they tend to differ from other, common, nontraumatic collapses, such as those from heart disease, EHS, or asthma.[6] Some players say that symptoms begin with leg and/or low-back pain and weakness, whereas others refer to "cramps that spread up my body." Some complain of weakness more than pain, and say legs "got wobbly, like Jello," whereas others say "I just don't feel right," or "these cramps are killing me." Some stoic players will stop running abruptly and either sit or lie down, saying "I can't go on," or "my legs won't go." Athletes may slouch and assume a position on their hands and knees, very anxious, with striking tachypnea. The instinctual wisdom to stop has likely saved the lives of many athletes with SCT. The telltale features of exertional sickling collapse are listed in **Box 3**.

Debate on Screening for SCT

Many debate screening. Some favor no screening and only the use of universal precautions, claiming this approach works for the Army; and yet, sickling deaths continue to occur in the Army, as recruits perform timed 2-mile runs.[33] Therefore, others favor screening with tailored precautions. Currently, all 50 states screen newborns to both facilitate education of parents by pediatricians on the potential risks for a child with SCT, and to attest to the SCT status during preparticipation physical evaluation for sports.

Tailored precautions seem preferable for college football. A questionnaire survey of NCAA Division-1 universities in 2006 found that approximately half were screening at least some athletes for SCT.[34] A recent lawsuit was the impetus for the NCAA, starting in 2010, to mandate SCT screening for all Division-1 athletes, unless they provide proof of prior screening or "opt out" of screening by signing a waiver. This landmark NCAA decision has been critiqued extensively, and the debate continues.[2]

Prevention and Treatment of Exertional Sickling Collapse

Exertional sickling collapse is a *medical emergency*. Tips for both prevention and treatment are listed in **Box 4**. Recommended precautions are based on evidence that sickling collapse is caused by the "perfect storm"—a lethal combination of unnecessary, maximal exertion, sustained for at least a few minutes, during a "heroic" effort that exceeds the physical limits of an athlete with SCT.

The game of football is composed of brief bursts of maximal activity with relatively prolonged periods of rest. Contrary to common wisdom, conditioning for NCAA Division-1 football has evolved in the opposite direction, with sustained bouts of maximal activity and only brief periods of rest between bouts. Some conditioning drills, for example, 16 to 24 successive 100-yard sprints, are unreasonable for the physiology of the sport.[35] In turn, irrational, intense conditioning for a game increases risk for poor outcomes in healthy athletes with SCT.

Box 3
Telltale features of exertional sickling collapse

- Dissimilar to heat cramps, muscle weakness exceeds muscle pain
- Athletes typically "slump" to the ground, unlike a "sudden fall" from cardiac pathology or the "hobble" from heat cramps
- Athletes are initially communicative, distinct from the unconscious state from a grave cardiac arrhythmia
- Muscles typically look and feel normal to the examiner, unlike "locked up" musculature from heat cramps
- Rapid tachypnea from lactic acidosis, yet pulmonary examination reveals good air movement, unlike an asthma attack
- Rectal temperature usually <103°F, as compared with temperatures typically >106°F in heat stroke

---

Box 4
Tips for prevention and treatment of exertional sickling collapse

Prevention

- Ideally, athletes with SCT should be allowed to set their "own pace"
- Gradual "build up" in training, with "paced progressions" and longer "rest spells"
- No extreme performance tests
- No "all-out" exertion sustained for >2–3 minutes
- Adjust for heat and altitude, control asthma, hydrate well, and disqualify from workouts during illnesses
- Set "tone" early, and educate athlete to discontinue exercise following "earliest, undue symptom" and have staff treat athlete as a case of "exertional sickling"

Treatment

- Monitor vital signs
- Give supplemental oxygen by face mask
- Cool athlete as necessary
- Failing immediate improvement, call 911, start intravenous line, prepare for cardiopulmonary resuscitation
- Rush athlete to hospital and tell physicians to anticipate explosive rhabdomyolysis

---

LUMBAR PARASPINAL MYONECROSIS

Compartment syndrome of the lower extremity can present clinically with exertional sickling collapse syndrome, both in the military and in college football.[36,37] Recently, lumbar paraspinal myonecrosis, a new variant of compartment syndrome, has been associated with exertional sickling in football. Notably, this syndrome is not unique to football or to athletes with SCT. It has been reported in skiers and in a waterskier, yet we believe that it may occur more often in football players with SCT.

In a retrospective review over a decade, we reported 4 cases of this syndrome among 13 college football players with SCT. The most severe occurred immediately after a drill that included pushing a weighted sled in a "bear-crawl" stance. All 4 had acute low-back pain and prolonged symptoms that limited practice for 1 to 2 weeks. Creatine kinase was elevated in all 4 cases, with the highest level 55,400 IU/L. Three of these cases had computed tomography and/or magnetic resonance imaging scans that documented muscle damage, including myonecrosis in the lumbar paraspinal musculature. All 4 athletes returned to play with training modifications.[38] One player had 3 recurrent episodes, 2 of them after college.

Another case was recently reported in a college lineman who developed symptoms 45 minutes after the commencement of a "one-on-one" contact drill. He was hospitalized for 2 weeks with paraspinal lumbar myonecrosis and was disqualified from football for several months.[39] Thus, lumbar paraspinal myonecrosis should be considered in the differential diagnosis when a player with SCT acutely develops severe low-back pain.

SPLENIC INFARCTION

Exertional sickling was a newsmaker in the autumn 2009, when Pittsburgh Steelers safety Ryan Clark, who has SCT, was told by his coach to skip the game against the Broncos in the mile-high altitude of Denver.[40] After Clark played in Denver in

2005, he was diagnosed with a "splenic contusion." Subsequently, he played in Denver in 2007, and suffered a sickling splenic infarction, developed an abscess in the necrotic spleen, and had splenectomy and cholecystectomy, which sidelined him for the remainder of that season.

Assuming that SCT is confined only to African American individuals can potentially lead to diagnostic errors, for example, when a white individual unaccustomed to altitude develops left lower chest or left upper quadrant (LUQ) pain while hiking, skiing, lifting weights, playing basketball, or even fishing.[41,42] A benchmark article reported 6 non-black men with "splenic syndromes" at mountainous altitudes. Four had exercised before the onset of severe LUQ pain. Spleen scans showed low uptake with or without clear-cut infarctions. Fortunately, none of them needed splenectomy. This risk may begin at 5000 ft and increases at higher altitudes.[43]

Another report of splenic syndrome in SCT details 4 patients who developed LUQ pain, nausea, vomiting, and respiratory splinting when exercising between 5500 and 12,000 ft. One was a white female physician skiing at 10,500 ft who was initially thought to have a pneumothorax.[44] In other cases, initial working diagnoses have included pleurisy, "side stitch," gastroenteritis, renal colic, or bowel obstruction.

Splenic infarction can also pose logistical problems for medical staff during "away games," as illustrated in the case of a basketball player from Alabama who suffered a splenic infarction while practicing for a game in Wyoming. He was sent to an emergency room and diagnosed with gastroenteritis twice in a span of 2 days. During the third hospital visit, he was correctly diagnosed with sickling splenic infarction, spent 3 days in a Laramie hospital, and subsequently flew home with supplemental oxygen while on the plane.[45]

By one tally, including 1 new case in a young white male trekker,[46] 30 of 50 reported SCT splenic infarctions at altitude were in non-black persons.[41] This may be partly an artifact both from vacation habits and reporting bias, yet one trekking company currently screens all clients for SCT.[46] The moral therefore should be: "Think of SCT splenic infarction in *anyone* who develops these clinical features at altitude. Diagnosed early, it responds to conservative therapy, including *descent*."

The pathophysiology of splenic infarction at altitude involves hypoxic sickling in the meandering circulation of the spleen. The fact that most cases reported were performing either mild or moderate, or vigorous "stop-and-go" exercise, with adequate time to "unsickle" during periods of rest, may explain why they suffered only splenic infarctions, not an exertional sickling collapse. A plausible explanation may be that even at altitude, it takes maximal exertion sustained for at least a few minutes to suffer an exertional sickling collapse. And last, autopsies from several football players who died from exertional sickling collapse have shown enlarged spleens congested with sickle cells, a possible prelude to splenic infarction.

HEMATURIA AND HYPOSTHENURIA

Gross hematuria is another complication of SCT, as described in a black junior college basketball player after a strenuous drill. Hematuria waxed and waned and resolved in 2 weeks. Past medical history had revealed a similar episode 5 years earlier. Intravenous pyelogram and cystoscopy results were normal and his hematuria was attributed to SCT.[47] The author has been queried about 2 other SCT athletes with gross hematuria, one a football player and the other a basketball player. In each case, the bleeding stopped within 2 weeks.

Gross hematuria results from sickling deep within the renal medulla, is occasionally associated with papillary necrosis,[48] and 80% is from the left kidney. It also can occur in white persons with SCT.[49] Gross hematuria occurs in fewer than 5% of persons with SCT lifelong. In some cases, comorbidity includes von Willebrand disease.[50] Rarely, bleeding can be massive, with passage of clots and advent of anemia.[48]

Initial therapy is conservative, including relative rest, hydration (mainly to avoid ureteral clots), and iron supplementation as needed. For progressive, persistent hematuria, there are several therapies, including vasopressin, epsilon-amino caproic acid, and balloon tamponade, yet there are no controlled trials that have evaluated the efficacy. Partial nephrectomy is a "last resort" therapy.[48] In most cases, with only conservative therapy, bleeding stops and the athlete returns to play.

Hyposthenuria, the inability to fully concentrate urine, is, in all probability, not a clinical problem for either high school or college athletes with SCT. It is true that because of sickling and altered blood flow through the vasa recta of the renal medulla, SCT carriers tend to develop hyposthenuria with advancing age; yet, we have not found this to be a problem in college athletes with SCT, and experts characterize hyposthenuria as "rarely clinically serious."[51]

In a recent study of men and women without SCT, urine osmolality increased to 800 to 1000 mOsm/kg H2O after an overnight (8 hours) period of water deprivation.[52] In a study of middle-aged subjects with SCT, after overnight water deprivation, urine osmolality ranged from about 500 to 800 mOsm/kg H2O; and, those with coexisting alpha-thalassemia trait had more concentrated urine than those without.[51] Overall, this seems a mild defect in concentrating ability, and it would likely be even milder in young athletes with SCT. It is possible that in some extreme combat settings, dehydration from hyposthenuria may be a sickling risk for a soldier with SCT. However, during the "daily life" of a young athlete with SCT, hyposthenuria seems a trivial concern.

VENOUS THROMBOEMBOLISM

In a retrospective study of approximately 65,000 consecutively hospitalized black men, pulmonary embolism was found in 2.2% of those with SCT versus 1.5% of those with normal hemoglobin, a relative risk of about 1.5.[53] As the researchers noted, this result must be regarded with caution because the difference was small and surrogate markers were used for the diagnosis of pulmonary embolism.

A new study, however, seems to confirm this risk. In a case-control study that compared 515 hospitalized black patients to 555 black controls attending medical clinics, the risk of venous thromboembolism was about twofold higher for those with SCT.[54] This increased risk was noticed for idiopathic and confirmed venous thromboembolism, in addition to first and recurrent episodes. An interesting paradox, however, was that although pulmonary embolism risk was increased approximately fourfold in those with SCT, the risk of deep venous thrombosis (without pulmonary embolism) was not meaningfully increased. Therefore, whether or not SCT increases the risk of venous thromboembolism remains unresolved and more research is needed.

This topic is critically important, because much too often we hear a report of an athlete who suffered a fatal pulmonary embolism, often after an injury that necessitated either immobilization or casting. Long, drawn-out plane or car trips can also pose a clotting problem for athletes.[55] A follow-up to the aforementioned case-control study has shown a tendency, albeit nonsignificant, for a higher risk of venous thromboembolism among black women with SCT who use oral contraceptives.[56] This research is clearly inconclusive. Yet, team physicians may consider monitoring athletes with SCT who have immobilizing injuries, especially those on oral contraceptives, for early signs of deep venous thrombosis, which may be a precursor to life-threatening pulmonary emboli.

SICKLING HEMOGLOBINOPATHIES

Few, if any, athletes with sickle cell anemia are able to compete on teams either in high school or beyond. Accordingly, the foremost sickling hemoglobinopathies that concern athletes are hemoglobin SC, S-beta-thalassemia, and hemoglobin SE. All 3 tend to cause a mild or moderate anemia that limits athletic stamina, along with other sickling problems, including occasional painful sickling crises and various splenic syndromes, especially at high altitudes or on plane flights. On first examination, it seems to be a medical paradox that hemoglobin SC induces so many sickling problems, despite being a hybrid of SCT and hemoglobin C trait, both of which are mostly benign medical conditions in everyday life. The explanation for this paradox is that hemoglobin C, by dehydrating the SC red blood cell, enhances the pathogenicity of hemoglobin S.

The author is familiar with several athletes with hemoglobin SC or S-beta-thalassemia who played football or basketball in high school; and, perhaps, there are many more cases that are unnoticed or unreported. In college, possibly because of more intense training and competition as compared with high school, relatively few athletes with these sickling hemoglobinopathies become known, or at least few are reported in the medical literature. However, in recent years, the author knows of 5 college athletes with sickling hemoglobinopathies, mostly via personal communications.

The first was a football player with hemoglobin SC who was initially not cleared by 2 universities, yet was accepted by a third. He suffered a total splenic infarction after weight lifting in training and dropped out of football. His case was reported in the literature.[57] The second was a female basketball player with hemoglobin SC who got through a college career despite suffering acute splenic pain during her first workout. The third was a fullback with S-beta-thalassemia who finished his college career; however, had limited stamina and was used primarily for short runs near the goal line. The fourth was a punter with hemoglobin SC who had prior, small splenic infarctions and occasional mild painful sickling crises, as well as splenic pain on plane flights. He got through 2 years of college football by using supplemental oxygen on team plane flights. The fifth athlete was a junior college basketball player with hemoglobin SC with prior splenic infarction on a plane flight, who completed his career with few problems, yet played only sparingly.

Finally, a youth football player aged 12, with hemoglobin SE, collapsed and died of exertional sickling in his first football practice in 2006.[10] He inherited the hemoglobin S from his black father and the hemoglobin E from his mother, who was from Thailand. Hemoglobin SE typically has about 60% to 65% hemoglobin S in each red blood cell, so it is similar to S-beta-thalassemia in severity.[58] In light of our increasing global society, we may see even more cases of hemoglobin SE in athletes.

SUMMARY

The foremost among sickle cell considerations in athletes is SCT, which can pose a range of clinical problems. The vital concern is exertional sickling collapse, which can be fatal, occurs in a variety of sports, and is a leading cause of death in college football. The chronology of sickling pathophysiology parallels the timing of exertional collapse. Recent research sheds light on the microcirculatory problems and adaptations in athletes with SCT. Sickling collapse is an "intensity"-associated syndrome that differs from the other common causes of collapse. Screening for SCT is a debated topic. The best approach in college football may be tailored precautions to prevent sickling collapse and enable athletes with SCT to thrive. Other clinical concerns in SCT are compartment syndromes and lumbar myonecrosis, splenic infarction, gross hematuria, hyposthenuria, and venous thromboembolism. Practical information on these concerns has been discussed, along with clinical pointers and experiences in athletes with sickling hemoglobinopathies more serious than SCT.

REFERENCES

1. Satterfield L, Ordine B. Field is goal. Kenwood's Gregory stuns medical experts by playing football varsity. Baltimore (MD): Sun; 2006.
2. Bonham VL, Dover GJ, Brody LC. Screening student athletes for sickle cell trait—a social and clinical experiment. N Engl J Med 2010;363:997–9.
3. Kark JA, Ward FT. Exercise and hemoglobin S. Semin Hematol 1994;31: 181–225.
4. Witt G. Autopsy shows A&T athlete had sickle cell blood trait. News-Record October 14, 2010.
5. Eichner ER. Sickle cell trait. J Sport Rehabil 2007;16:197–203.
6. Eichner ER. Sickle cell trait in sports. Curr Sports Med Rep 2010;9:347–51.
7. Pretzlaff RK. Death of an adolescent athlete with sickle cell trait caused by exertional heat stroke. Pediatr Crit Care Med 2002;3:308–10.
8. Wright R. Time to Cisti and make up. ABQ Journal 2006.
9. Eichner ER. Sickle cell trait, exercise, and altitude. Phys Sportsmed 1986;14(11): 144–57.
10. Graham K. Blood disorder blamed in death. St Petersburg Times; 2006.
11. Jones SR, Binder RA. Sudden death in sickle-cell trait. N Engl J Med 1970;282: 323–5.
12. Diggs LW. The sickle cell trait in relation to the training and assignment of duties in the Armed Forces: III. Hyposthenuria, hematuria, sudden death, rhabdomyolysis, and acute tubular necrosis. Aviat Space Environ Med 1984; 55:358–64.
13. Koppes GM, Daly JJ, Coltman CA Jr, et al. Exertion-induced rhabdomyolysis with acute renal failure and disseminated intravascular coagulation in sickle cell trait. Am J Med 1977;63:313–7.
14. Kark JA, Posey DM, Schumacher HR. Sickle-cell trait as a risk factor for sudden death in physical training. N Engl J Med 1987;317:781–7.
15. Kark JA. Sickle cell trait. Available at. http://sickle.bwh.harvard.edu/sickle_trait.html. Accessed November 7, 2009.
16. Scoville SL. Recruit mortality. In: DeKoning BL, editor. Recruit medicine. Washington, DC: Defense Department, Army, Borden Institute. Walter Reed Army Medical Center; 2006. p. 519–53.
17. Schrier RW, Henderson HS, Tisher CC, et al. Nephropathy associated with heat stress and exercise. Ann Intern Med 1967;67:356–76.
18. Gardner JW, Kark JA. Fatal rhabdomyolysis presenting as mild heat illness in military training. Mil Med 1994;159:160–3.
19. Anzalone ML, Green VS, Buja M, et al. Sickle cell trait and fatal rhabdomyolysis in football training: a case study. Med Sci Sports Exerc 2010;42:3–7.
20. Osnes J-B, Hermansen L. Acid-base balance after maximal exercise of short duration. J Appl Physiol 1972;32:59–62.
21. Hartley LH, Vogel JA, Landowne M. Central, femoral, and brachial circulation during exercise in hypoxia. J Appl Physiol 1973;34:87–90.

22. Medbo JI, Sejersted OM. Acid-base and electrolyte balance after exhausting exercise in endurance-trained and sprint-trained subjects. Acta Physiol Scand 1985;125:97–109.
23. Bergeron MF, Cannon JG, Hall EL, et al. Erythrocyte sickling during exercise and thermal stress. Clin J Sport Med 2004;14:354–6.
24. Martin TW, Weisman IM, Zeballos RJ. Exercise and hypoxia increase sickling in venous blood from an exercising limb in individuals with sickle cell trait. Am J Med 1989;87:48–55.
25. Monchanin G, Connes P, Wouassi D, et al. Hemorheology, sickle cell trait, and alpha-thalassemia in athletes: effects of exercise. Med Sci Sports Exerc 2005; 37:1086–92.
26. Connes P, Sara F, Hardy-Dessources MD, et al. Effects of short supramaximal exercise on hemorheology in sickle cell trait carriers. Eur J Appl Physiol 2006; 97:143–50.
27. Monchanin G, Serpero LD, Connes P, et al. Effects of progressive and maximal exercise on plasma levels of adhesion molecules in athletes with sickle cell trait with or without alpha-thalassemia. J Appl Physiol 2007;102:169–73.
28. Tripette J, Loko G, Samb A, et al. Effects of hydration and dehydration on blood rheology in sickle cell trait carriers during exercise. Am J Physiol Heart Circ Physiol 2010;299:H908–14.
29. Vincent L, Feasson L, Oyone-Enguelle S, et al. Remodeling of skeletal muscle microvascular in sickle cell trait and alpha-thalassemia. Am J Physiol Heart Circ Physiol 2009;298:H375–84.
30. Vincent L, Feasson L, Oyono-Enguelle S, et al. Skeletal muscle structural and energetic characteristics in subjects with sickle cell trait, alpha-thalassemia, or dual hemoglobinopathy. J Appl Physiol 2010;109:728–34.
31. Connes P, Racinals S, Sara F, et al. Does the pattern of repeated sprint ability differ between sickle cell trait carriers and healthy subjects? Int J Sports Med 2006;27:1–6.
32. Aufradet E, Monchanin G, Oyonno-Engelle S, et al. Habitual physical activity and endothelial activation in sickle cell trait carriers. Med Sci Sports Exerc 2010;42: 1987–94.
33. Sanchez CE, Jordan KM. Exertional sickness. Am J Med 2010;123:27–30.
34. Clarke CE, Paul S, Stilson M, et al. Sickle cell trait preparticipation screening practices of collegiate physicians. Clin J Sport Med 2006;16:440a.
35. McGrew CA. NCAA football and conditioning drills. Curr Sports Med Rep 2010;6: 185–6.
36. Hieb LD, Alexander AH. Bilateral anterior and lateral compartment syndromes in a patient with sickle cell trait. Case report and review of the literature. Clin Orthop Relat Res 1988;228:190–3.
37. Schrotenboer B. Lineman collapsed in workout last month. Awareness spreading on "exertional sickling." San Diego (CA): Union Tribune; 2009.
38. Schnebel B, Eichner ER, Anderson S, et al. Sickle cell trait and lumbar myonec- rosis as a cause of low back pain in athletes. Med Sci Sports Exerc 2008; 40(Suppl 5):537a.
39. Hale MH, Prine BR, Clugston JR, et al. Severe low back pain in a football player. Poster presented at 17th annual AMSSM conference. Las Vegas, March 25–29, 2008.
40. Eichner ER. Exertional sickling. Curr Sports Med Rep 2010;9:3–4.
41. Eichner ER. Sickle cell trait in athletes: three clinical concerns. Curr Sports Med Rep 2007;6:134–5.

42. Tiernan CJ. Splenic crisis at high altitude in 2 white men with sickle cell trait. Ann Emerg Med 1999;33:230–3.
43. Lane PA, Githens JH. Splenic syndrome at mountain altitudes in sickle cell trait. Its occurrence in nonblack persons. JAMA 1985;253:2251–4.
44. Franklin QJ, Compeggie M. Splenic syndrome in sickle cell trait: four case presentations and a review of the literature. Mil Med 1999;164:230–3.
45. Ortega JO. Nausea, vomiting, and abdominal pain in a collegiate basketball player. Clin J Sport Med 2006;15:443a.
46. Hannaford M. A case of splenic infarction at high altitude in sickle cell trait by Dr Alison Cook. Available at: http://expeditionmedicine.wordpress.com. posted April 22, 2008. Accessed November 12, 2010.
47. Eichner ER. Hematuria—a diagnostic challenge. Phys Sportsmed 1990;18(11): 53–63.
48. Ataga KI, Orringer EP. Renal abnormalities in sickle cell disease. Am J Hematol 2000;63:205–21.
49. Oksenhendler E, Bourbigot B, Desbazeille F, et al. Recurrent hematuria in 4 white patients with sickle cell trait. J Urol 1984;132:1201–3.
50. Brody JI, Levison SP, Jung C-J. Sickle cell trait and hematuria associated with von Willebrand syndromes. Ann Intern Med 1977;86:529–33.
51. Gupta AK, Kirchner KA, Nicholson R, et al. Effects of alpha-thalassemia and sickle polymerization tendency on the urine-concentrating defect of individuals with sickle cell trait. J Clin Invest 1991;88:1963–8.
52. Hancock ML 2nd, Bichet DG, Eckert GJ, et al. Race, sex, and the regulation of urine osmolality: observations made during water deprivation. Am J Physiol Regul Integr Comp Physiol 2010;299:R977–80.
53. Heller P, Best WR, Nelson RB, et al. Clinical implications of sickle-cell trait and glucose-6-phosphate dehydrogenase deficiency in hospitalized black male patients. N Engl J Med 1979;300:1001–5.
54. Austin H, Key NS, Benson JM, et al. Sickle cell trait and the risk of venous thromboembolism among blacks. Blood 2007;110:908–12.
55. Eichner ER. Blood clots and plane flights. Curr Sports Med Rep 2009;8:106–7.
56. Austin H, Lally C, Benson JM, et al. Hormonal contraception, sickle cell trait, and risk for venous thromboembolism among African American women. Am J Obstet Gynecol 2009;200:620–3.
57. Ouyang DL, Kohrt HE, Garza D, et al. Massive splenic infarction in a collegiate football player with hemoglobin SC disease. Clin J Sport Med 2008;18:89–91.
58. Masiello D, Heeney MM, Adewoye AH, et al. Hemoglobin SE disease—a concise review. Am J Hematol 2007;82:643–9.

Advances in Management of the Female Athlete Triad and Eating Disorders

Karie N. Zach, MD[a,b], Ariane L. Smith Machin, PhD[c],
Anne Z. Hoch, DO[b,d],*

KEYWORDS

- Female athlete triad • Endothelial dysfunction • Folic acid
- Disordered eating

Since Congress passed Title IX in 1972, which ensured women would have equal opportunities for interscholastic sports participation in public institutions at the high school and college level, the number of females participating in athletics has increased dramatically. In 1971–1972, there were 3.7 million males participating in high school athletics, compared with 300,000 females. National data gathered for the 2009–2010 high school season noted 4.5 million males and 3.2 million females, which represents virtually a 1000% increase in female athletes.[1] A similar trend has also been observed at the collegiate level. Among Division I, II, and III schools, the number of female athletes grew from 74,000 in 1982 to 178,000 athletes in 2008, an increase of 140%.[2]

There are numerous potential benefits for women who participate in athletics. Female athletes have been shown to have higher self-esteem, better grades, higher graduation rates, less depression, have lower rates of teen pregnancy, and engage less in "high-risk behaviors," such as drug use.[3] However, secondary to a complex combination of endocrine and metabolic factors, female athletes are at risk for a serious health concern: the female athlete triad (triad). The purpose of this article

There was no funding needed to support this work.
The authors have no financial disclosure.
[a] Department of Orthopaedic Surgery, Sports Medicine Center, Medical College of Wisconsin, 8700 Watertown Plank Road, Milwaukee, WI 53226, USA
[b] Department of Physical Medicine and Rehabilitation, Medical College of Wisconsin, 8700 Watertown Plank Road, Milwaukee, WI 53226, USA
[c] Women's Sports Medicine Program, Sports Medicine Center, Medical College of Wisconsin, 8700 Watertown Plank Road, Milwaukee, WI 53226, USA
[d] Women's Sports Medicine Program, Department of Orthopaedic Surgery, Sports Medicine Center, Medical College of Wisconsin, 8700 Watertown Plank Road, Milwaukee, WI 53226, USA
* Corresponding author. Department of Orthopaedic Surgery, Sports Medicine Center, Medical College of Wisconsin, 8700 Watertown Plank Road, Milwaukee, WI 53226.
E-mail address: azeni@mcw.edu

Clin Sports Med 30 (2011) 551–573
doi:10.1016/j.csm.2011.03.005
0278-5919/11/$ – see front matter © 2011 Elsevier Inc. All rights reserved.

is to provide an update on new issues related to management of the triad, including the relationship between athletic-associated amenorrhea and endothelial dysfunction, the role of optimizing energy availability within the context of disordered eating, amenorrhea, and bone density, and therapeutic approaches to individual, group-based, and pharmacologic interventions.

HISTORY OF THE FEMALE ATHLETE TRIAD

In June 1992, the American College of Sports Medicine (ACSM) convened a panel of experts to address a set of disorders observed in adolescent and young adult female athletes: disordered eating, amenorrhea, and osteoporosis.[4] In 1997, the ACSM position statement defined the triad, and identified the population at risk and the need to screen female athletes.[5] Subsequently, 10 years later, directed by the plethora of research in this area, the ACSM updated its definition of the triad. The 2007 position statement defines the triad as a spectrum of interrelationships among energy availability, menstrual function, and bone mineral density (BMD), which may have clinical manifestations including eating disorders, functional hypothalamic amenorrhea, and osteoporosis. Athletes are distributed along a spectrum between health and disease (**Fig. 1**). The ideal female athlete is to the far right of the spectrum, which defines optimal health. The athlete may fall anywhere along the spectrum, and medical interventions should not be deferred until the athlete has reached the far left of the spectrum, which defines "significant pathology." In the 2007 ACSM position statement, a new consequence of athletic associated amenorrhea, impaired endothelium-dependent arterial vasodilation, was introduced, which is discussed in the endothelial dysfunction section elsewhere in this article.[6,7]

Energy availability refers to a spectrum of eating issues that ranges from optimal energy availability to low energy availability, with or with an eating disorder.[6] Energy availability, based on the work of Loucks, is defined as the amount of "unused" dietary energy remaining after exercise training for all other metabolic processes.[8] Athletic amenorrhea was changed to include a spectrum of menstrual function ranging from eumenorrhea to amenorrhea, including oligomenorrhea, luteal deficiency, and anovulation.[6] The definition of primary amenorrhea was reduced from 16 to 15 years.[9]

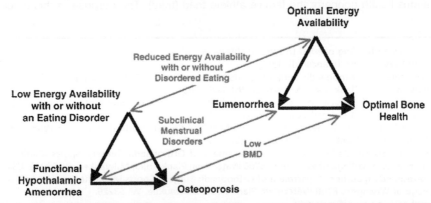

Fig. 1. The female athlete triad: energy availability, menstrual function, and bone mineral density. A spectrum of health and disease. (*From* Nattiv A, Loucks AB, Manore MM, et al. American College of Sports Medicine position stand. The female athlete triad. Med Sci Sports Exerc 2007;39(10):1868; with permission.)

Significant changes were also introduced to elucidate the third component of the triad, osteoporosis. The 1997 ACSM position statement used the World Health Organization (WHO) criteria for diagnosing osteopenia and osteoporosis. Numerous studies have established the WHO criteria for fracture risk in postmenopausal women, but assessing the impact of low bone mass on fracture risk to other populations is problematic,[10] primarily because there is no established standard to adjust for bone size, pubertal stage, skeletal maturity, or body composition.[6] The 2007 ACSM statement incorporated the International Society for Clinical Densitometry (ISCD) recommendations, that BMD in premenopausal women and children be expressed as z scores, to compare individuals to age-matched and sex-matched controls.[11,12] z Scores below −2.0 are defined as "low bone density below the expected range for age" in premenopausal women, and as "low bone density for chronologic age" in children.[11,12] The ISCD also recommends an established diagnosis of osteoporosis at z score of less than −2.0 and the presence of secondary clinical risk factors including either amenorrhea, eating disorders, hyperparathyroidism, or glucocorticoid exposure. Because athletes participating in weight-bearing sports typically have 5% to 15% higher BMD than nonathletes,[13–17] the ACSM recommends further clinical investigation for a BMD z score of less than −1.0 in an athlete.[6]

PREVALENCE OF THE FEMALE ATHLETE TRIAD

Recently, numerous studies have offered insightful information and have documented the prevalence of the triad at various competition levels (**Table 1**). Despite increased awareness and meaningful research, the triad is highly prevalent in athletes. However, varying methodology used in these studies to classify disordered eating, menstrual dysfunction, and low BMD precludes meaningful comparisons.

At the high school level, one study showed that 78% of varsity female athletes had one or more components of the triad, and 50% reported menstrual dysfunction.[18] In another study of high school athletes, 18.2%, 23.5%, and 21.8% met criteria for disordered eating, menstrual irregularity, and low bone mass, respectively.[19] By comparison, both these studies found that a lower percentage of subjects had all 3 criteria (1% and 1.2%, respectively).[18,19] In Division II collegiate female athletes from 7 different sports, Beals and Hill[20] found 25% of athletes with disordered eating, 26% with menstrual dysfunction, and 10% with low BMD, with a z score of less than −1.0. Similar to the studies in high school athletes, only 2.6% had all 3 components of the triad.

Among young Turkish athletes between 16 and 25 years of age in 10 sports, Vardar and colleagues[21] found a prevalence rate of 1.36%. In female runners between 18 and 25 years of age, Cobb and colleagues[22] reported that 36% met criteria for abnormal menses; those runners with menstrual dysfunction had lower BMD than eumenorrheic runners, and there was an association with disordered eating and menstrual dysfunction. In a study of recreational female triathletes, 60% had at least one component of the triad.[23] Torstveit and Sundgot-Borgen[24] found that 4.3% of elite Norwegian athletes had evidence of all 3 components, with 60% classified as "at risk" for the triad. In Brazilian elite swimmers, 47% had at least one of the components and 1.3% had all 3 components of the triad.[25] Finally, a recent study[26] in 2011 of professional ballet dancers reported a 14% prevalence of the triad and impaired brachial artery vasodilation. Of significant concern, 64% of the dancers had evidence of endothelial dysfunction.

ENDOTHELIAL DYSFUNCTION

The triad of low energy availability, menstrual dysfunction, and low BMD in females is well documented in the literature. There is increasing evidence for a potential fourth

Table 1
Female athlete triad prevalence studies: methodology

Study	Population	Disordered Eating	Menstrual Dysfunction	Bone Mineral Density
Nicols[19] 2006	High school athletes	EDE-Q	1° Amen = 16 y; 2° Amen ≥3 mo; Oligo >35 d	z score <−1, <−2
Hoch et al,[18] 2009	High school athletes	EAT-26, 3-day food for EA	1° Amen = 15 y old; 2° Amen >3 cycles; Oligo >35 d	z score <−1
Cobb et al,[22] 2003	Runners 18–26 y	EDI-DT, EDI-BD, EDI-BT	Amenorrhea/Oligo 0–9 menses/year	g/cm^2, no T or z score
Beals and Hill[20] 2006	College athletes; 7 sports	Selected questions from EDI, EDE-Q	1° Amen = 16 y old; 2° Amen >3 cycles, <12 cycles in 12 mo, <6 cycles in 6 mo, >10 d variation in cycle	z score <−1, <−2
Vardar et al,[21] 2005	Turkish athletes 16–25 y; 10 sports	EAT-40	1° Amen = 16 y old; 2° Amen >3 cycles; Oligo >35 d	T score <−1[a]
Torstveit and Sundgot-Borgen[24] 2005	Elite Norwegian athletes 13–39 y	EDI-DT, EDI-BD, selected questions, interview	1° Amen = 16 y old; 2° Amen >3 cycles; Oligo >35 d; short luteal <22 d	z score <−1
Schtscherbyna et al,[25] 2009	Elite Brazilian swimmers 11–19 y	EAT-26, BITE, BSQ	1° Amen = 16 y old; 2° Amen >6 mo or period = 3 cycles; Oligo >35 d	z score <−2
Hoch et al,[23] 2007	Triathletes	EAT-26, 3-day food for REE	History of amenorrhea	T and z score
Hoch et al,[26] 2011	Professional ballet dancers	EDE-Q, 3-day food for EA	1° Amen = 15 y old; 2° Amen >3 cycles; Oligo >35 d	z score <−1

Abbreviations: 1° Amen, primary amenorrhea; 2° Amen, secondary amenorrhea; BITE, Bulimic Investigatory Test Edinburgh; BSQ, Body Shape Questionnaire; EA, energy availability; EAT-26, 26-item Eating Attitudes Test; EAT-40, 40-item Eating Attitudes Test; EDE-Q, Eating Disorder Examination Questionnaire; EDI-BD, Body Dissatisfaction subscale of the Eating Disorder Inventory; EDI-BT, Bulimic Tendencies subscale of the Eating Disorder Inventory; EDI-DT, Drive for Thinness subscale of the Eating Disorder Inventory; REE, resting energy expenditure; Oligo, oligomenorrhea.
[a] Only patients with disordered eating and menstrual dysfunction had bone mineral testing done.

component, endothelial dysfunction—a well-established "sentinel" event in the pathogenesis of cardiovascular disease.[27] In addition, cardiovascular disease is the number one cause of death in women.[28] Therefore, early detection of endothelial dysfunction and appropriate, timely therapeutic interventions for the triad are cornerstones of long-term health and longevity in young athletic women with amenorrhea.

The techniques used for assessment of coronary reactivity are invasive and expensive, and not ideal for clinical purposes, especially if serial measurements are required. An alternative approach is to noninvasively examine vascular function in a peripheral vessel, sustaining the belief and understanding that vascular disease is a systemic process.[29,30] The gold standard for noninvasive assessment of endothelial function is brachial ultrasound scanning.[31] High-resolution ultrasonography can easily be used to assess flow-mediated dilation (FMD) of the brachial artery. Brachial artery diameter and flow velocity are measured both at baseline and following induction of reactive hyperemia by forearm occlusion using a blood pressure cuff.[32] Athletes with normal endothelial function typically show an increase in diameter in the range of 5% to 15%.[33] The authors endorse this is as a valid technique, because several studies have shown a positive relationship between brachial artery endothelial dysfunction and coronary artery endothelial dysfunction.

Anderson and colleagues[34] demonstrated a close relation between coronary artery endothelium-dependent vasomotor responses to acetylcholine and FMD in the brachial artery. The positive predictive value of abnormal brachial dilation in predicting coronary endothelial dysfunction was 95%. In a study by Neunteufl and colleagues,[35] FMD of the brachial artery was significantly impaired in patients with coronary artery disease (CAD) compared with controls. Lieberman and colleagues[36] reported that FMD of the brachial artery was significantly lower in young adults (<40 years old) who showed angiographic evidence of CAD, as compared with FMD in age-matched healthy controls.

In turn, the association between brachial artery endothelial dysfunction and coronary artery endothelial dysfunction is important, because coronary artery endothelial dysfunction has been shown to correlate with cardiovascular events. For example, Schachinger and colleagues[37] noted a greater incidence of cardiovascular events (death, unstable angina, myocardial infarction, ischemic stroke) in patients with impaired coronary function. Suwaidi and colleagues[38] noted no cardiac events (cardiac death, myocardial infarction, revascularization) in patients with normal or mild coronary endothelial dysfunction, compared with a cardiac event rate of 14% in those with severe coronary endothelial dysfunction. Moreover, similar findings by Halcox and colleagues[39] and Targonski and colleagues[40] identified that coronary endothelial dysfunction is independently associated with an increased risk of cardiovascular events.

A few important studies document a detrimental relationship between athletic amenorrhea and brachial artery endothelial dysfunction. Hoch and colleagues[41] studied 32 female collegiate athletes who ran at least 25 miles per week. Baseline brachial artery diameters were similar among amenorrheic, oligomenorrheic, and control groups. However, brachial artery FMD was significantly lower in amenorrheic athletes (1.08% ± 0.91%) compared with the oligomenorrheic athletes (6.44% ± 1.28%) and the control group (6.38% ± 1.38%). Rickenlund and colleagues[42] noted similar results, with a significant decrease in FMD of the brachial artery in amenorrheic endurance athletes compared with oligomenorrheic and eumenorrheic athletes.

Finally, a strong case for routine assessment of FMD may be made based on the data from the recent 2011 study on professional ballet dancers, 64% of whom had decreased FMD of the brachial artery. Of the ballet dancers with decreased FMD,

72% reported menstrual dysfunction, 14% had been treated with oral contraceptive (OC) therapy secondary to amenorrhea, and 14% were eumenorrheic. There was no suitable explanation for decreased FMD in the eumenorrheic dancers, and it was beyond the scope of that study to determine whether they were ovulatory.[26] Possible explanations include nutritional deficiencies or decreased aerobic fitness. Nevertheless, this study showed correlations both between abnormal FMD and estrogen levels, and abnormal FMD and low BMD (**Fig. 2**). These correlates are important because currently, FMD testing is not performed routinely. It must be noted that there were important limitations to the aforementioned studies that included only a small, "select" population of athletes, and large-scale studies are needed for further evaluation.

TREATMENT OF ENDOTHELIAL DYSFUNCTION IN THE FEMALE ATHLETE

Studies have examined the potential for treating impaired FMD. In men, regular aerobic exercise has been shown to restore endothelial-dependent vasodilation.[43–45] The mechanism of improved endothelial dysfunction is thought to be partially due to increased nitric oxide (NO) bioavailability.[33] In female athletes, Rickenlund and colleagues[46] demonstrated significantly increased FMD after 9 months of treatment with a low-dose, monophasic combined OC (30 μg ethinyl estradiol and 150 μg levonorgestrel). FMD in amenorrheic endurance athletes increased from 1.42% ± 0.98% before OC treatment to 4.88% ± 2.2% after OC therapy. This finding demonstrates that OC therapy can potentially restore impaired endothelial function mediated via the protective effects of estrogen.

However, in 2002 the Women's Health Initiative (WHI) study found a 22% increased risk of cardiovascular events in postmenopausal women using hormone replacement therapy that included both estrogen and progestin.[47] In addition, a recent 2010 follow-up study of the WHI trial published in the *Journal of the American Medical Association* noted increased incidence of breast cancer and breast cancer mortality in postmenopausal women treated with estrogen and progestin.[48] Therefore, although this risk has been described in postmenopausal women, alternative therapeutic interventions to restore endothelial function must be investigated in young athletes.

Folic acid supplementation is a potential option for treatment. Folates have been suggested to contribute to the endogenous regeneration of tetrahydrobiopterin, an essential cofactor for endothelial NO synthase production,[49] which may result in increased NO production following daily supplementation (**Fig. 3**). In vitro data suggest a direct antioxidant effect of folates on vasculature,[50] thereby increasing NO bioavailability and improving FMD.[51] There have been numerous, small-scale studies that have documented improvement of endothelium-dependent vasodilation with folic acid supplementation.

Folic acid has been documented to improve endothelium-dependent vasodilation in men with hypertension, CAD, congestive heart failure, diabetes mellitus type 2, hyperhomocystinemia, and peripheral vascular disease.[52–58] These studies suggest that in these patient populations, high-dose folic acid may offer vasculoprotective effects. There have been several recent studies on "select" female athlete populations noting improved FMD after folic acid supplementation (**Table 2**). Hoch and colleagues[59] showed that folic acid supplementation, 10 mg/d for 4 to 6 weeks, significantly improved brachial artery FMD in eumenorrheic women runners when compared with a placebo, control group. A separate study by Hoch and colleagues[60] in amenorrheic female runners noted improvement of brachial artery FMD after 4 weeks of folic acid supplementation at a dose of 10 mg/d. A more recent study in female ballet

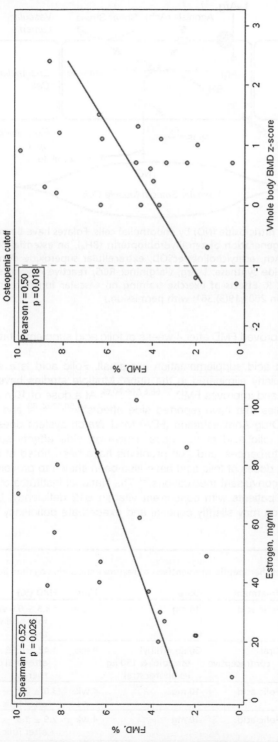

Fig. 2. Correlation between abnormal FMD (%) and estrogen and whole-body BMD z score. (*From* Hoch AZ, Papanek P, Szabo A, et al. Association between the female triad athlete and endothelial dysfunction in dancers. Clin J Sport Med 2011;21(1):123; with permission.)

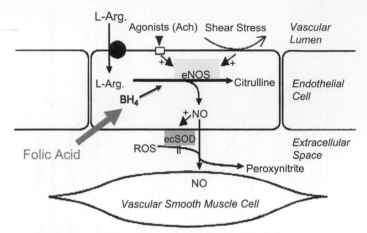

Fig. 3. Production of nitric oxide (NO) by endothelial cells. Folates have been suggested to participate in the regeneration of tetrahydrobiopterin (BH_4), an essential cofactor in the production of NO. Ach, acetylcholine; ecSOD, extracellular superoxide dismutase; eNOS, endothelial nitric oxide synthase; L-Arg, L-arginine; ROS, reactive oxygen species. (*From* Gielen S, Hambrecht R. Effects of exercise training on vascular function and myocardial perfusion. Cardiol Clin 2001;19(3):361; with permission.)

dancers showed improved FMD after 4 weeks of folic acid supplementation at a dose of 10 mg/d.[61]

The risks of folic acid supplementation are small. Folic acid is a water-soluble vitamin that is regularly eliminated in the urine. Multiple studies have shown that 10 mg daily is safe and improves FMD.[54,56,57,59,60,62] At a dose of 10 mg daily, there have been no studies that have reported side effects[54,56,57,62,63] and significantly, the US Food and Drug Administration (FDA) Med Watch system does not list any adverse effects of folic acid at this dose. However, side effects such as upset stomach, sleep disturbances, and skin problems have been noted at doses higher than 15 mg/d. High doses of folic acid have also been shown to provoke seizures in patients taking anticonvulsant medications.[64] The National Institutes of Health have advised caution in patients with concurrent vitamin B12 deficiency, because folic acid supplementation may silently conceal and exacerbate deficiency.[65] Moreover,

Table 2
Small-scale studies of therapeutic interventions to restore endothelial dysfunction in females

Patients	Treatment	Dose	Time	FMD (%)
Eumenorrheic runners[59]	Folic acid	10 mg	4–6 wk	↑3.5 ± 0.6 vs ↑0.1 ± 0.2 folic acid vs placebo therapy
Amenorrheic endurance athletes[46]	Oral contraceptive	30 μg ethinyl estradiol & 150 μg levonorgestrel	9 mo	1.42 ± 0.98 → 4.88 ± 2.2 after oral contraceptive therapy
Amenorrheic runners[60]	Folic acid	10 mg	4 wk	3.0 ± 2.3 → 7.7 ± 4.5 after folic acid therapy
Professional ballet dancers[61]	Folic acid	10 mg	4 wk	2.9 ± 1.5 → 7.1 ± 2.3 after folic acid therapy

a recent study suggested that folic acid supplementation may increase the risk of colorectal adenoma in patients with a known history of colorectal adenomas.[66] Despite potential side effects at higher doses, the prospective benefits from low-dose folic acid supplementation in athletes may outweigh the risks, especially in athletes opposed to estrogen supplementation. Clinicians could potentially recommend folic acid on a daily basis to athletes with endothelial dysfunction; however, large-scale studies are needed to accurately determine the lowest efficacious dose and optimal duration of treatment.

Disordered Eating: Energy Availability

Treatment of the triad often involves a multidisciplinary team approach including a sports physician, registered sports dietician, certified sports psychologist and, optimally, family, coaches, and friends. The main focus of treatment is to remedy low energy availability and provide emotional support, which can be an especially challenging task if an athlete has a concomitant eating disorder. The first step is to meet with a sports dietician who is familiar with the clinical implications of the triad and is knowledgable with calculating energy availability. "Energy availability" is defined as the amount of dietary energy remaining for other bodily functions after exercise training.[6,8,10] The gold-standard approach is to have the athlete fill out a 3-day food diary, including 2 weekdays and 1 weekend day, and to weigh food portions.[67] The dietician should always review proper meal portion sizes before the athletes record food weight. During this period, the athlete can also wear an accelerometer to determine how many calories are being expended. Subsequently, the dietician can use the food record and accelerometer data to appropriately calculate energy availability and formulate a meal plan to accurately correct low energy availability.

Support for a causal relationship between energy availability and menstrual cycles was provided by Williams and colleagues,[68] who demonstrated that in exercising monkeys, amenorrhea could be reversed by increasing food intake while maintaining a daily training program. If the energetics of the restoration of menstrual cycle in monkeys holds true for women who are undergoing equivalent training, an approximately 20% increase in calories would lead to ovulation in about 2 months, and a 50% increase in calories would lead to ovulation in about 2 weeks.[69] In a study of 100 adolescent girls with anorexia nervosa, 86% of patients resumed menses within 6 months after increasing their weight to 90% of standard body weight.[70]

In addition to reversal of low energy availability and amenorrhea, adequate calcium and vitamin D supplementation, and weight training are effective therapies for the third component of the triad, low BMD. A case report by Fredericson and Kent[71] showed a significant increase in BMD in a female athlete after gaining weight. This finding is encouraging because it contradicts the concept that low BMD is irreversible in adolescents and young athletes. Weight-training programs have been shown to increase BMD, and should be implemented in all athletes with low BMD.[72] Antiresorptive therapies, for example, bisphosphonates, have not been tested and are not approved by the FDA in younger patients with low BMD. The use of bisphosphonates is controversial is this population secondary to their potential for teratogenicity. Furthermore, bisphosphonates can linger in mineralized bone for several years.[73]

EATING DISORDERS

Sport participation for the female athlete has become a possible risk factor for developing an eating disorder.[74–77] In a survey of National Collegiate Athletic Association (NCAA) institutions, Dick[78] found that 93% of the reports from athletic directors indicated that eating disorders occurred among their female athletes. Eating disorders may increase the risk of depressive disorders, anxiety disorders, substance abuse, and health problems.[79] Furthermore, eating disorders can increase distress and functional impairment, as well as inpatient hospitalization, suicide attempts, and mortality.[80–83] Because of these potentially negative, long-term consequences, it is imperative that thorough and expeditious treatment be available and readily accessible to athletes.

Advances in Multidisciplinary Team Approach

An approach to the treatment and management of symptoms of eating disorders involves the use of a multidisciplinary team (team). The method was initially recommended as a primary way to manage athletes with symptoms of eating disorders more than 20 years ago,[84] and while this approach is largely unchanged, the complexity and degree of involvement of individuals has changed.[85] It has been suggested that the team should consist of a broader range of individuals, including coaches, athletic trainers, team physicians, sport dieticians, sport psychologists, and perhaps sports administrators.[86] Bonci and colleagues[86] also suggest that registered sports dieticians should have an expertise in treating the athletic population. Moreover, the ACSM 2007 position statement emphasized that the first goal of treatment should be to increase energy availability by increasing energy intake and/or reducing energy expenditure.[6]

Thompson and Sherman[85] have suggested several considerations while assembling a team. First, the sports medicine physician should be the main coordinator for the athlete's care. Second, the physician determines the degree of involvement of each team member and ensures that his or her contribution is therapeutic. Third, each of the team members must operate within acceptable ethical guidelines.[87] The team should be used for a variety of roles and needs to be aware of the various aspects of the treatment process. The team should have a strategy for approaching high-risk or symptomatic athletes, and recognize that the timing of the therapeutic approach to an athlete is a pivotal component of good care.[85] The team members should have a good relationship with the athlete, or at least be comfortable discussing sensitive and important issues.[88] Members of the team should also work together to address standards for safely returning the athlete to participation, adequately monitor symptoms and therapeutic strategies, and potential communication with teammates and the media.[85]

Trattner-Sherman and Thompson[87] recommend declaring the athlete "injured" and treating the athlete with an eating disorder akin to an athlete with a physical injury, which would typically prevent athletic participation. Confidentiality must not be compromised unless the athlete has explicitly agreed to communicate with all members of the team. In addition, the athlete should be informed regarding scheduled meetings of the multidisciplinary team to discuss their progress and/or evaluation of therapy.[89] During the management process, it may be helpful to generate a "contract" that outlines clear and concrete expectations that will need to be accomplished by the athlete before returning to sports participation. This agreement would help eliminate ambiguity about the recovery process and create leverage for the athlete to be motivated to engage in healthier behaviors.

Advances in Psychotherapy

It is imperative that the clinician treating the individual has special expertise and knowledge regarding the athletic population, as there are many unique aspects to sport that need to be considered and managed. While the athlete is working with the multidisciplinary team, he or she may use individual therapy, group therapy, or pharmacotherapy, and may be hospitalized depending on the severity of symptoms. Individual therapy is one of the most common treatment approaches, as this provides an opportunity to gain both a greater understanding of the psychological roots of eating disorders and whether the eating disorder predated the athlete's involvement in athletics. In addition, psychotherapy is helpful for the athlete to learn more effective coping strategies (eg, relaxation techniques, assertiveness training, identifying and modifying negative thinking patterns), manage eating-disorder symptoms (eg, identify "risky" moods or situations, learn how to engage in alternative behaviors, engage in self-monitoring), and possibly restore weight while alleviating the anxiety that can surround this phase of treatment.

Cognitive-behavioral treatment (CBT) for eating disorders is currently considered to be the most effective treatment, especially for bulimia. CBT incorporates a broad range of treatment approaches, but most are conceptualized using Beck's cognitive therapy.[90] In CBT, a client undergoes approximately 20 treatment sessions with a focus on 3 major stages.[91] The main goals include normalization of eating, reducing attempts to diet, eliminating binge eating and purging, and altering beliefs, thoughts, and values that maintain the patterns of disordered eating.[92] For example, in one phase of treatment athletes would be asked to identify thoughts immediately preceding an identified event or trigger (eg, eating a particular type of food, not engaging in regular exercise) and create counterstatements that would oppose their automatic thoughts that they could use to manage some of the intense and maladaptive thought patterns that contribute to the maintenance of unhealthy attitudes and behaviors. This same treatment approach can be used for those experiencing symptoms of anorexia, with only minor variation and typically an extended time frame.

Despite the potential advantages of CBT,[93–95] other studies have suggested that CBT is unsupportive for about 50% of treated individuals.[95,96] Therefore, researchers have proposed that comorbidity with other disorders and other factors related to the athlete may contribute to therapeutic effectiveness. For example, CBT directly attempts to change the content of maladaptive eating-related cognitions[97]; however, some of the egosyntonic cognitions associated with eating disorders can be resistant to direct modification efforts.[98] Consequently, new approaches to treatments for eating disorders have been investigated.

A more recent intervention, acceptance and commitment therapy (ACT),[99,100] relies on the premise that a client's reaction to a thought or feeling is changeable, but that the internal experience is unaffected. ACT attempts to teach clients how to be more accepting of distressing cognitions and feelings because attempting to control unwanted experiences is often ineffective and occasionally may prove to be counterproductive.[101] A treatment protocol for eating disorders has been developed and applied,[102] and the two central components of ACT, mindfulness and acceptance, are associated with better treatment outcomes in eating disorders.[103,104] Another reason why ACT might be particularly useful for the treatment of eating pathology relates to the treatment process of identifying and clarifying individuals' ultimate life values. By helping identify core values and broader goals emanating from them (eg, achieve pregnancy in the future), ACT helps clients to both reorient toward more meaningful activities and to become more willing to tolerate internal discomfort for the sake of what they identify as "truly important."[92]

In addition to CBT and ACT, dialectical behavior therapy (DBT)[105] has also received attention for its promising results. DBT, a cognitive-behavioral treatment originally developed for women with borderline personality disorder, is a comprehensive, multimodal, skills-based treatment that balances behavioral strategies with acceptance-based strategies and targets life-threatening, therapy-interfering, and quality-of-life interfering behaviors.[106] During treatment, DBT addresses deficits in interpersonal relationships, affect regulation, and impulse control. Although DBT has been very helpful for individuals who have been diagnosed with an eating disorder and concurrent disorder (such as borderline personality disorder), researchers have suggested that DBT is effective for those without Axis II pathology.[107] For example, researchers have postulated that eating pathology represents a maladaptive method to regulate negative affect,[108,109] and that the techniques within DBT can assist in reducing symptoms of eating disorders. In one study, Safer and colleagues[109] applied DBT to individuals diagnosed with binge and purge behaviors, and found that 28.6% were abstinent from binge eating and purging behaviors as opposed to zero participants in the wait-list control condition.

Finally, enhanced cognitive behavioral therapy (CBT-E) is a transdiagnostic approach applicable to all types of eating disorders, though modifications are made for significantly underweight individuals. Fairburn[110] developed two forms of CBT-E; one focuses solely on eating disorders, whereas the other explores low self-esteem and extreme perfectionism issues. Although CBT-E is based on a cognitive-behavioral approach, it does not place as much importance on traditional CBT methods such as formal thought records, cognitive restructuring, Socratic reasoning, and formal behavioral experiments. Instead, the treatment explores the commonly encountered traits of clinical perfectionism, core low self-esteem, and interpersonal difficulties. These components are important to address because if they are not resolved, an individual may be more resistant to treatment and experience a relapse of eating-disorder symptoms.[111] In one study, Fairburn and colleagues[112] found that the majority of patients (n = 154) responded rapidly to CBT-E, and the changes were sustained over the following year, the time at which relapse is most likely to occur. Approximately two-thirds of those who completed treatment had a complete and lasting response, with many of the remainder showing substantial improvement. To date, there have not been any studies investigating CBT-E within the athlete population. It would be helpful to continue to investigate the effectiveness of this approach within this population, as it seems to be a promising treatment protocol for the management of all eating disorders.

Advances in Pharmacotherapy

Although several psychotherapies have been shown to be effective in reducing eating and associated psychopathology,[93] growing research suggests that pharmacotherapies[93,113,114] may also be effective, and can be an adjunct to, traditional therapy. Selective serotonin-reuptake inhibitor (SSRI) antidepressants,[115] antiepileptic drugs,[116,117] the selective norepinephrine reuptake inhibitor atomoxetine,[118] the atypical antipsychotic olanzapine (Zyprexa)[119] and antiobesity medications[120–122] have all shown promise in reducing a variety of symptoms of eating disorders. However, among the drug treatments, SSRIs (Paxil and so forth) are the first-line treatments of choice, especially in primary care,[123] and may be a good initial option if an athlete presents with symptoms of disordered eating. The scope of this article does not allow all details to be provided regarding all uses and research in anorexia, bulimia, and binge-eating disorder. For more information regarding pharmacotherapy with anorexic patients, refer to Crow and colleagues,[124] Pike and colleagues,[125] or Zhu and Walsh.[126] For an in-depth review of pharmacotherapy research with bulimic patients, refer to Mitchell and colleagues[96] or Zhu and Walsh.[126] As a general guideline, when incorporating pharmacotherapy with athletes it is important to be aware of the level of competition, and the possible ban on various substances by different governing bodies within the athletic context.[127] The NCAA[128] indicates that there is no complete list of banned drug examples. Athletes are therefore advised and encouraged to check and review, with their athletic department medical staff, the labels of all products, medications, and/or supplements prior to consumption.

Advances in Intervention Programs

Whereas individual therapy typically affects the individual in treatment, prevention and intervention programs aim to target and modify attitudes and behavior within a larger group setting. Initial prevention programs for eating disorders consisted primarily of didactic psychoeducation, and were usually directed toward adolescents.[129,130] The rationale of these programs was that information about the adverse effects of eating disorders would prevent individuals from using maladaptive methods as a means of weight control.[131] For example, most programs taught students about natural changes in body composition associated with physical maturation, and encouraged development of a positive body image.

Although the first phase of intervention programs had good intentions, they were not entirely effective in reducing eating pathology.[131] Therefore, the second phase of eating-disorder prevention programs were developed. These programs were also didactic in format, and included additional information on resisting the sociocultural pressures of thinness and suggestions for healthy-weight–control methods.[132] These programs were developed under the pretext that sociocultural pressures were extremely important in the development of eating disorders, and that extreme dieting and compensatory behaviors emerged as a result of trying to meet "appropriate" cultural standards of weight. For instance, these programs included components that aimed to facilitate knowledge, to resist negative media images about eating and "body image," and to develop coping skills to resist sociocultural pressures regarding thinness and dieting.

Recently, the prevention programs have targeted high-risk populations, using interactive groups focusing on risk factors that have been researched as predictors of eating disorders.[131] The effects of these programs offered to high-risk individuals have been shown to be more effective than universal programs offered to all available participants.[133] It has been hypothesized that the individuals with initially prominent symptoms may be more willing to integrate themselves into therapeutic eating-disorder programs, enhancing the desired effects.[134] These individuals may be experiencing more distress, motivating them to become actively engaged in the program. In addition, the interactive programs are more likely to involve exercises that allow participants to apply the skills taught in the intervention, which may increase skill acquisition.[131]

Athletes Targeting Healthy Exercise and Nutrition Alternatives (ATHENA) is a universal, selective program for middle and high school sport participants that is scripted, coach facilitated, and peer led.[135] The program was created to decrease risk factors for eating disorders and the use of diet and performance-enhancing drugs. The curriculum includes components to build skills to control mood, counter media influences, and provide information on sports nutrition and strength training. In addition, information is presented on factors that contribute to the risk of disordered eating and the use of body-shaping drugs. The curriculum was provided to sports teams in small groups led by an assigned peer leader in 8 45-minute sessions. Although the ATHENA program initially showed significant decreases in the targeted risk factors and reduced the ongoing and new use of body-shaping substances,[135] 1 to 3 years later athletes did not show continued reductions in eating pathology.[136]

Table 3
Advances in individual and group-based psychological interventions for athletes with eating disorders and symptoms of the triad

Therapy	Empirical Support	Theoretical Underpinnings	Athlete Application
Cognitive-Behavioral Therapy (CBT); Beck[141] 1970	Brownley et al,[93] 2007 Shapiro et al,[94] 2007 Wilson et al,[95] 2007	Focuses on identifying and modifying thoughts, emotions, and behaviors; focuses on the present; can be brief or long term	Gains an awareness of automatic thoughts, mood shifts, and behaviors that are affecting food choices, body image distortions, and ability to maintain weight
Acceptance and Commitment Therapy (ACT); Hayes and Wilson[99], 1994	Heffner et al,[102] 2002 Baer et al,[103] 2005 Kristeller et al,[104] 2006	Uses mindfulness and acceptance strategies; observing and experiencing versus directly trying to deliberately modify negative thoughts, emotions, or behaviors	Begins to "just notice," accept, and embrace uncomfortable or negative thoughts/emotions toward food, eating, or body size and shape
Dialectical Behavioral Therapy (DBT); Linehan[105] 1993	Safer et al,[109] 2001 Telch et al,[142] 2001 Ben-Porath et al,[143] 2009	Targets emotional regulation by teaching adaptive skills to foster self-monitoring, regulation of emotions, and distress tolerance; emphasizes acceptance, change, and mindful awareness	Observes their emotional regulation cycle and patterns, understands and accepts environmental or personal cues that impact mood, disordered eating, or body distortions; take action
Enhanced Cognitive Behavioral Therapy (CBT-E); Fairburn[110] 2008	Fairburn et al,[112] 2009	Offers two approaches, one focusing on eating disorders and the other exploring low self-esteem and perfectionism; uses a highly structured yet personalized approach to tackling core dysfunctional beliefs and eating behavior	Identifies underlying thought processes and personality characteristics contributing to the development and maintenance of disordered eating, and explores the impact of these variables on self-esteem, mood, and interpersonal relationships
Dissonance-Based Prevention (DBP); Stice et al,[137] 2008	Matusek et al,[144] 2004 Green et al,[145] 2005 Becker et al,[146] 2008 Becker et al,[139] 2010	Attempts to elicit inconsistencies between eating and body size/shape attitudes and behaviors through activities, discussion, and participating in body activism; develops healthier attitudes and behaviors by conclusion of group	Identifies and discusses cultural and sport-specific body ideals, recognizes how participating in this dynamic has emotional and physical costs, identifies alternative attitudes and behaviors, participates in body activism, and practices resisting ideals

Another approach that has generated some positive findings among eating-disorder symptoms involves dissonance-based prevention programming.[137] The dissonance-based approach attempts to elicit inconsistencies between attitudes and behaviors through various activities and discussions, with the ultimate intention of reestablishing a "new" consistency that is congruent with healthier and more adaptive functioning. For example, participants will take a stand against the socioculturally prescribed "thin-ideal" and engage in other acts of activism (eg, identifying behaviors previously deemed "unacceptable," such as wearing shorts, and engaging in this behavior at least once) which, according to dissonance theory, will begin to influence their behaviors to be more congruent with their new attitudinal change.

The Female Athlete Body Project is a multiyear program based on the work by Stice and colleagues[138] that uses a cognitive-dissonance approach for the prevention of eating disorders within the athlete population. The program was peer led and occurred in 3 sessions of 75 to 80 minutes. Topics included definitions of the sport-specific and athlete-specific thin ideal, factors that enhance sport performance, and the female athlete triad. Results suggest that participants experienced significant decreases in the thin-ideal internalization, negative affect, eating pathology, and body dissatisfaction post treatment, and that those changes were maintained at 6-week follow-ups for all measures except thin-ideal internalization.

Further, Becker and colleagues[139] pilot-tested the effectiveness of an athlete-modified peer-led version of dissonance-based prevention and healthy-weight intervention at reducing eating-disorder risk factors in female college athletes. In their study, 157 student athletes representing 9 varsity sport teams at a Division III University were enrolled. The program consisted of two phases: the first phase consisted of the participation in the Female Athlete Body Project, and in the second phase participants were randomly assigned to the dissonance-based or healthy-weight–based interventions. Significant, positive findings in both the dissonance and healthy-weight groups included reductions in thin-ideal internalization, dietary restraint, bulimic pathology, shape and weight concern, negative affect at 6 weeks, bulimic pathology, shape concern, and negative affect at 1-year follow-up. In addition, the investigators suggested that the use of the Female Athlete Body Project led to a noticeable increase in students spontaneously seeking medical consultation for the triad.

Thus these recent interventions that focus on specific risk factors for eating disorders will be more effective than those that focus on nonestablished risk factors.[133] Specifically, programs that focus on increasing resistance to sociocultural pressures for thinness, body satisfaction, self-esteem, and healthy-weight management skills cause greater and more positive behavioral and attitudinal changes than those that consist of only psychoeducation or use variables that are not established eating-disorder risk factors, such as stress and coping skills.[140] Specific information regarding each therapeutic approach and applications to athletes are shown in **Table 3**. It is imperative that researchers continue investigating promising programs, as there is a major lack of research and interventions specifically designed for the unique needs of the athlete population.

SUMMARY

While the prevalence of all 3 components of the triad is low in female athlete populations, there is a much higher risk of having at least one of the components. One can argue that having just one component of the triad is a red flag that needs to be addressed to prevent the other 2 components. It is extremely challenging to compare prevalence studies, as each study uses different methodological tools for screening.

As a general recommendation, there should be a consensus on which screening tools to use for disordered-eating menstrual dysfunction, and on reporting low BMD for research purposes. Endothelial dysfunction is a potential fourth component, which is concerning for future cardiovascular risk, public health issues, and athletic performance. Folic acid should be considered a potential safe and inexpensive therapeutic treatment to restore endothelial-dependent vasodilation, although the optimal dosage and length of treatment is yet to be defined. There are various options for treating disordered eating in the athletic population, including a multidisciplinary team that can treat low energy availability. Athletes are owed a "duty of care," and high schools, colleges, universities, and various athlete-focused clinics should develop and offer a comprehensive education and treatment program that includes education, screening, an intervention protocol, and a treatment plan. Consistent school policies to protect the athlete are also needed.

ACKNOWLEDGMENTS

The authors would like to thank Karen Gonzalez, BS, MS, for her editorial expertise.

REFERENCES

1. NFSHSA. 2009–10 high school athletics participation survey: based on competition at the high school level in 2009–10 school year. In: The National Federation of States High Schools Association handbook. Kansas City (MO): National Federation of State High Schools; 2010. p. 51–2.
2. DeHaas DM. NCAA sports sponsorship and participation rates report 1981–1982, 2007–2008. 2009. Available at: http://www.ncaapublications.com/productdownloads/PR2009.pdf. Accessed March 12, 2011.
3. Lopiano D. Gender equity in sports. In: Agostini R, editor. Medical and orthopedic issues of active and athletic women. Philadelphia: Hanley & Belfus; 1994. p. 13–22.
4. Yeager KK, Agostini R, Nattiv A, et al. The female athlete triad: disordered eating, amenorrhea, osteoporosis. Med Sci Sports Exerc 1993;25(7):775–7.
5. Otis CL, Drinkwater B, Johnson M, et al. American College of Sports Medicine position stand. The female athlete triad. Med Sci Sports Exerc 1997;29(5): 1669–71.
6. Nattiv A, Loucks AB, Manore MM, et al. American College of Sports Medicine position stand. The female athlete triad. Med Sci Sports Exerc 2007;39(10): 1867–82.
7. Beals KA, Meyer NL. Female athlete triad update. Clin Sports Med 2007;26(1): 69–89.
8. Loucks AB. Low energy availability in the marathon and other endurance sports. Sports Med 2007;37(4/5):348–52.
9. Practice Committee of the American Society for Reproductive Medicine. Current evaluation of amenorrhea. Fertil Steril 2004;82(1):266–72.
10. Leib ES. Treatment of low bone mass in premenopausal women: when may it be appropriate? Curr Osteoporos Rep 2005;3(1):13–8.
11. Writing Group for the ISCD Position Development Conference. Diagnosis of osteoporosis in men, premenopausal women, and children. J Clin Densitom 2004;7(1):17–26.
12. Leslie WD, Adler RA, El Hajj FG, et al. Application of the 1994 WHO classification to populations other than postmenopausal Caucasian women: the 2005 ISCD official positions. J Clin Densitom 2006;9(1):22–30.

13. Lebrun CM. The female athlete triad: what's a doctor to do? Curr Sports Med Rep 2007;6:397–404.
14. Dook JE, James C, Henderson NK, et al. Exercise and bone mineral density in mature female athletes. Med Sci Sports Exerc 1997;29(3):291–6.
15. To WW, Wong MW, Lam IY. Bone mineral density differences between adolescent dancers and non-exercising adolescent females. J Pediatr Adolesc Gynecol 2005;18(5):337–42.
16. Cassell C, Benedict M, Specker B. Bone mineral density in elite 7- to 9-yr-old female gymnasts and swimmers. Med Sci Sports Exerc 1996;28(10):1243–6.
17. Nickols-Richardson SM, Modlesky CM, O'Connor PJ, et al. Premenarcheal gymnasts possess higher bone mineral density than controls. Med Sci Sports Exerc 2000;32(1):63–9.
18. Hoch AZ, Pajewski NM, Moraski L, et al. Prevalence of the female athlete triad in high school athletes and sedentary students. Clin J Sport Med 2009;19(5): 421–8.
19. Nichols JF, Rauh MJ, Lawson MJ, et al. Prevalence of the female athlete triad syndrome among high school athletes. Arch Pediatr Adolesc Med 2006; 160(2):137–42.
20. Beals KA, Hill AK. The prevalence of disordered eating, menstrual dysfunction, and low bone mineral density among US collegiate athletes. Int J Sport Nutr Exerc Metab 2006;16(1):1–23.
21. Vardar S, Vardar E, Altun G, et al. Prevalence of the female athlete triad in Endirne, Turkey. J Sports Sci Med 2005;4:550–5.
22. Cobb KL, Bachrach LK, Greendale G, et al. Disordered eating, menstrual irregularity, and bone mineral density in female runners. Med Sci Sports Exerc 2003; 35(5):711–9.
23. Hoch AZ, Stavrakos JE, Schimke JE. Prevalence of female athlete triad characteristics in club triathlon team. Arch Phys Med Rehabil 2007;88(5):681–2.
24. Torstveit MK, Sundgot-Borgen J. The female athlete triad exists in both elite athletes and controls. Med Sci Sports Exerc 2005;37(9):1449–59.
25. Schtscherbyna A, Soares E, de Oliveira F, et al. Female athlete triad in elite swimmers of the city of Rio de Janeiro, Brazil. Nutrition 2009;25(6):634–9.
26. Hoch AZ, Papanek P, Szabo A, et al. Association between the female triad athlete and endothelial dysfunction in dancers. Clin J Sport Med 2011;21(1): 119–25.
27. Ross R. The pathogenesis of atherosclerosis: a perspective for the 1990s. Nature 1993;362(6423):801–9.
28. NCHS. Health data interactive: centers for disease control and prevention. WISQARS leading causes of death reports, 1999–2006. AHA Heart Disease and Stroke Statistics 2010. Available at: http://www.cdc.gov/nchs/fastats/ deaths.htm. Accessed March 12, 2011.
29. Ross R. Atherosclerosis: current understanding of mechanisms and future strategies in therapy. Transplant Proc 1993;25(2):2041–3.
30. Ross R. Atherosclerosis—an inflammatory disease. N Engl J Med 1999;340(2): 115–26.
31. Thijssen DH, Black MA, Pyke KE, et al. Assessment of flow mediated dilation (FMD) in humans: a methodological and technical guideline. Am J Physiol Heart Circ Physiol 2011;300(1):H2–12.
32. Celermajer DS, Sorensen KE, Gooch VM, et al. Non-invasive detection of endothelial dysfunction in children and adults at risk of atherosclerosis. Lancet 1992; 340(8828):1111–5.

33. Walther C, Gielen S, Hambrecht R. The effect of exercise training on endothelial function in cardiovascular disease in humans. Exerc Sport Sci Rev 2004;32(4): 129–34.

34. Anderson TJ, Uehata A, Gerhard MD, et al. Close relation of endothelial function in the human coronary and peripheral circulations. J Am Coll Cardiol 1995;26(5): 1235–41.

35. Neunteufl T, Katzenschlager R, Hassan A, et al. Systemic endothelial dysfunction is related to the extent and severity of coronary artery disease. Atherosclerosis 1997;129(1):111–8.

36. Lieberman EH, Gerhard MD, Uehata A, et al. Flow-induced vasodilation of the human brachial artery is impaired in patients <40 years of age with coronary artery disease. Am J Cardiol 1996;78:1210–4.

37. Schachinger V, Britten MB, Zeiher AM. Prognostic impact of coronary vasodilator dysfunction on adverse long- term outcome of coronary heart disease. Circulation 2000;101(16):1899–906.

38. Suwaidi JA, Hamasaki S, Higano ST, et al. Long-term follow-up of patients with mild coronary artery disease and endothelial dysfunction. Circulation 2000; 101(9):948–54.

39. Halcox JP, Schenke WH, Zalos G, et al. Prognostic value of coronary vascular endothelial dysfunction. Circulation 2002;106(6):653–8.

40. Targonski PV, Bonetti PO, Pumper GM, et al. Coronary endothelial dysfunction is associated with an increased risk of cerebrovascular events. Circulation 2003; 107(22):2805–9.

41. Hoch AZ, Dempsey RL, Carrera GF, et al. Is there an association between athletic amenorrhea and endothelial cell dysfunction? Med Sci Sports Exerc 2003;35(3):377–83.

42. Rickenlund A, Eriksson MJ, Schenck-Gustafsson K, et al. Amenorrhea in female athletes is associated with endothelial dysfunction and unfavorable lipid profile. J Clin Endocrinol Metab 2005;90(3):1354–9.

43. Higashi Y, Sasaki S, Kurisu S, et al. Regular aerobic exercise augments endothelium-dependent vascular relaxation in normotensive as well as hypertensive subjects: role of endothelium-derived nitric oxide. Circulation 1999; 100(11):1194–202.

44. DeSouza CA, Shapiro LF, Clevenger CM, et al. Regular aerobic exercise prevents and restores age-related declines in endothelium-dependent vasodilation in healthy men. Circulation 2000;102(12):1351–7.

45. Donato AJ, Uberoi A, Bailey DM, et al. Exercise-induced brachial artery vasodilation: effects of antioxidants and exercise training in elderly men. Am J Physiol Heart Circ Physiol 2010;298(2):H671–8.

46. Rickenlund A, Eriksson MJ, Schenck-Gustafsson K, et al. Oral contraceptives improve endothelial function in amenorrheic athletes. J Clin Endocrinol Metab 2005;90(6):3162–7.

47. Rossouw JE, Anderson GL, Prentice RL, et al. Risks and benefits of estrogen plus progestin in healthy postmenopausal women: principal results from the Women's Health Initiative randomized controlled trial. JAMA 2002;288(3):321–33.

48. Chlebowski RT, Anderson GL, Gass M, et al. Estrogen plus progestin and breast cancer incidence and mortality in postmenopausal women. JAMA 2010; 304(15):1684–92.

49. Wever RM, van Dam T, van Rijn HJ, et al. Tetrahydrobiopterin regulates superoxide and nitric oxide generation by recombinant endothelial nitric oxide synthase. Biochem Biophys Res Commun 1997;237(2):340–4.

50. Verhaar MC, Wever RM, Kastelein JJ, et al. 5-Methyltetrahydrofolate, the active form of folic acid, restores endothelial function in familial hypercholesterolemia. Circulation 1998;97(3):237–41.
51. Bonetti PO, Lerman LO, Lerman A. Endothelial dysfunction: a marker of atherosclerotic risk. Arterioscler Thromb Vasc Biol 2003;23(2):168–75.
52. Verhaar MC, Wever RM, Kastelein JJ, et al. Effects of oral folic acid supplementation on endothelial function in familial hypercholesterolemia: a randomized placebo-controlled trial [In Process Citation]. Circulation 1999;100:335–8.
53. Maxwell AJ, Anderson BE, Cooke JP. Nutritional therapy for peripheral arterial disease: a double-blind, placebo-controlled, randomized trial of HeartBar. Vasc Med 2000;5(1):11–9.
54. Wilmink HW, Stroes ES, Erkelens WD, et al. Influence of folic acid on postprandial endothelial dysfunction. Arterioscler Thromb Vasc Biol 2000;20(1):185–8.
55. Title LM, Cummings PM, Giddens K, et al. Effect of folic acid and antioxidant vitamins on endothelial dysfunction in patients with coronary artery disease. J Am Coll Cardiol 2000;36(3):758–65.
56. Title LM, Ur E, Giddens K, et al. Folic acid improves endothelial dysfunction in type 2 diabetes—an effect independent of homocysteine-lowering. Vasc Med 2006;11(2):101–9.
57. Moens AL, Claeys MJ, Wuyts FL, et al. Effect of folic acid on endothelial function following acute myocardial infarction. Am J Cardiol 2007;99(4):476–81.
58. Woo KS, Chook P, Chan LL, et al. Long-term improvement in homocysteine levels and arterial endothelial function after 1-year folic acid supplementation. Am J Med 2002;112(7):535–9.
59. Hoch AZ, Pajewski NM, Hoffmann RG, et al. Possible relationship of folic acid supplementation and improved flow-mediated dilation in premenopausal, eumenorrheic athletic women. Am J Sports Med 2009;8:123–9.
60. Hoch AZ, Lynch SL, Jurva JW, et al. Folic acid supplementation improves vascular function in amenorrheic runners. Clin J Sport Med 2010;20(3):205–10.
61. Hoch AZ, Papanek P, Havlik HS, et al. Prevalence of the female athlete triad/tetrad in professional ballet dancers. Med Sci Sports Exerc 2009;41(5):524.
62. Woo KS, Chook P, Lolin YI, et al. Folic acid improves arterial endothelial function in adults with hyperhomocystinemia. J Am Coll Cardiol 1999;34(7):2002–6.
63. US Food and Drug Administration. The FDA safety information and adverse event reporting program: medical product safety information. Available at: http://www.fda.gov/medwatch/SAFETY.htm. Accessed November 20, 2010.
64. Herbert V. Folic acid. In: Shils M, Olson J, Shike M, et al, editors. Modern nutrition in health and disease. Baltimore (MD): Williams & Wilkins; 1999. p. 433–66.
65. National Institutes of Health. National Institutes of Health, Office of Dietary Supplements. Dietary supplement fact sheet: folate. Available at: http://ods.od.nih.gov/factsheets/folate.asp#en10. Accessed November 19, 2010.
66. Cole BF, Baron JA, Sandler RS, et al. Folic acid for the prevention of colorectal adenomas: a randomized clinical trial. JAMA 2007;297(21):2351–9.
67. Biro G, Hulshof KF, Ovesen L, et al. Selection of methodology to assess food intake. Eur J Clin Nutr 2002;56(Suppl 2):S25–32.
68. Williams NI, Helmreich DL, Parfitt DB, et al. Evidence for a causal role of low energy availability in the induction of menstrual cycle disturbances during strenuous exercise training. J Clin Endocrinol Metab 2001;86(11):5184–93.
69. Williams NI. Lessons from experimental disruptions of the menstrual cycle in humans and monkeys. Med Sci Sports Exerc 2003;35(9):1564–72.

70. Golden NH, Jacobson MS, Schebendach J, et al. Resumption of menses in anorexia nervosa. Arch Pediatr Adolesc Med 1997;151(1):16–21.
71. Fredericson M, Kent K. Normalization of bone density in a previously amenorrheic runner with osteoporosis. Med Sci Sports Exerc 2005;37(9):1481–6.
72. Winters-Stone KM, Snow CM. Musculoskeletal response to exercise is greatest in women with low initial values. Med Sci Sports Exerc 2003;36(4):1691–6.
73. McNicholl DM, Heaney LG. The safety of bisphosphonate use in premenopausal women on corticosteroids. Curr Drug Saf 2010;5(2):182–7.
74. Hausenblas HA, Carron AV. Eating disorder indices and athletes: an integration. J Sport Exerc Psychol 1999;21:230–58.
75. Striegel-Moore RH, Silberstein LR, Rodin J. Toward an understanding of risk factors for bulimia. Am Psychol 1986;41(3):246–63.
76. Sundgot-Borgen J, Corbin C. Eating disorders among female athletes. Phys Sportsmed 1987;15(2):89–95.
77. Sundgot-Borgen J, Torstveit MK. Prevalence of eating disorders in elite athletes is higher than in the general population. Clin J Sport Med 2004;14(1):25–32.
78. Dick RW. Eating disorders in NCAA athletic programs. J Athl Train 1991;26: 136–40.
79. Johnson JG, Cohen P, Kasen S, et al. Eating disorders during adolescence and the risk for physical and mental disorders during early adulthood. Arch Gen Psychiatry 2002;59(6):545–52.
80. Patton GC, Selzer R, Coffey C, et al. Onset of adolescent eating disorders: population based cohort study over 3 years. BMJ 1999;318(7186):765–8.
81. Lewinsohn PM, Striegel-Moore RH, Seeley JR. Epidemiology and natural course of eating disorders in young women from adolescence to young adulthood. J Am Acad Child Adolesc Psychiatry 2000;39(10):1284–92.
82. Hoek HW, van Hoeken D. Review of the prevalence and incidence of eating disorders. Int J Eat Disord 2003;34(4):383–96.
83. Crow SJ, Peterson CB, Swanson SA, et al. Increased mortality in bulimia nervosa and other eating disorders. Am J Psychiatry 2009;166(12):1342–6.
84. Thompson RA. Management of the athlete with an eating disorder: implications for the sport management team. Sport Psychol 1987;1:114–26.
85. Thompson RA, Sherman R. Eating disorders in sport. New York: Routledge/ Taylor & Francis Group; 2010.
86. Bonci CM, Bonci LJ, Granger LR, et al. National Athletic Trainers' Association position statement: preventing, detecting, and managing disordered eating in athletes. J Athl Train 2008;43:80–108.
87. Trattner-Sherman R, Thompson RA. Athletes and disordered eating: four major issues for the professional psychologist. Prof Psychol Res Pr 2001;32(1): 27–33.
88. Managing student-athletes' mental health issues. Indianapolis (IN): National Collegiate Athletic Association; 2007.
89. Hildebrandt T. A review of eating disorders in athletes: recommendations for secondary school prevention and intervention programs. J Appl Sch Psychol 2005;21(2):145–67.
90. Forman E, Herbert J. New directions in cognitive behavior therapy: acceptance-based therapies. In: O'Donohue W, Fisher J, editors. General principles and empirically supported techniques of cognitive behavior therapy. Hoboken (NJ): John Wiley & Sons, Inc; 2009. p. 77–101.
91. Fairburn CG, Marcus M, Wilson G. Cognitive-behavioral therapy for binge eating and bulimia nervosa: a comprehensive treatment manual. In: Fairburn CG,

Wilson G, editors. Binge eating: Nature, assessment, and treatment. New York: Guilford Press; 1993. p. 361–404.

92. Juarascio AS, Forman EM, Herbert JD, et al. Acceptance and commitment therapy versus cognitive therapy for the treatment of comorbid eating pathology. Behav Modif 2010;34(2):175–90.

93. Brownley KA, Berkman ND, Sedway JA, et al. Binge eating disorder treatment: a systematic review of randomized controlled trials. Int J Eat Disord 2007;40(4): 337–48.

94. Shapiro JR, Berkman ND, Brownley KA, et al. Bulimia nervosa treatment: a systematic review of randomized controlled trials. Int J Eat Disord 2007; 40(4):321–36.

95. Wilson GT, Grilo CM, Vitousek KM. Classification of eating disorders: toward DSM-V. Int J Eat Disord 2007;40:S123–9.

96. Mitchell JE, Agras S, Wonderlich S. Treatment of bulimia nervosa: where are we and where are we going? Int J Eat Disord 2007;40(2):95–101.

97. Vanderlinden J. Many roads lead to Rome: why does cognitive behavioural therapy remain unsuccessful for many eating disorder patients? Eur Eat Disord Rev 2008;16(5):329–33.

98. Guarda AS. Treatment of anorexia nervosa: insights and obstacles. Physiol Behav 2008;94(1):113–20.

99. Hayes SC, Wilson KG. Acceptance and commitment therapy: altering the verbal support for experiential avoidance. Behav Anal 1994;17(2):289–303.

100. Hayes SC, Strosahl KD, Wilson KG. Acceptance and commitment therapy: an experiential approach to behavior change. New York: Guilford; 2003.

101. Hayes SC. Acceptance and commitment therapy, relational frame theory, and the third wave of behavior therapy. Behav Ther 2004;35:639–65.

102. Heffner M, Sperry J, Eifert GH, et al. Acceptance and commitment therapy in the treatment of an adolescent female with anorexia nervosa: a case example. Cognit Behav Pract 2002;9(3):232–6.

103. Baer R, Fischer S, Huss D. Mindfulness and acceptance in the treatment of disordered eating. J Ration Emot Cogn Behav Ther 2005;23(4):281–300.

104. Kristeller JL, Baer R, Quillian-Wolever R. Mindfulness-based approaches to eating disorders. In: Baer R, editor. Mindfulness-based treatment approaches. San Diego (CA): Elsevier; 2006. p. 75–91.

105. Linehan MM. Skills training manual for treating borderline personality disorder. New York: Guilford Press; 1993.

106. Chen EY, Matthews L, Allen C, et al. Dialectical behavior therapy for clients with binge-eating disorder or bulimia nervosa and borderline personality disorder. Int J Eat Disord 2008;41(6):505–12.

107. Ben Porath DD, Wisniewski L, Warren M. Differential treatment response for eating disordered patients with and without a comorbid borderline personality diagnosis using a dialectical behavior therapy (DBT)-informed approach. Eat Disord 2009;17(3):225–41.

108. Heatherton TF, Baumeister RF. Binge eating as escape from self-awareness. Psychol Bull 1991;110(1):86–108.

109. Safer DL, Telch CF, Agras WS. Dialectical behavior therapy for bulimia nervosa. Am J Psychiatry 2001;158(4):632–4.

110. Fairburn CG. Cognitive behavior therapy and eating disorders. New York: The Guilford Press; 2008.

111. Bissada H. Review of 'Cognitive behavior therapy and eating disorders'. Can J Psychiatry 2009;54(11):783–4.

112. Fairburn CG, Cooper Z, Doll HA, et al. Transdiagnostic cognitive-behavioral therapy for patients with eating disorders: a two-site trial with 60-week follow-up. Am J Psychiatry 2009;166(3):311–9.

113. Carter WP, Hudson JI, Lalonde JK, et al. Pharmacologic treatment of binge eating disorder. Int J Eat Disord 2003;34(S1):S74–88.

114. Stefano SC, Bacaltchuk J, Blay SL, et al. Antidepressants in short-term treatment of binge eating disorder: systematic review and meta-analysis. Eat Behav 2008;9(2):129–36.

115. Guerdjikova AI, McElroy SL, Kotwal R, et al. High-dose escitalopram in the treatment of binge-eating disorder with obesity: a placebo-controlled monotherapy trial. Hum Psychopharmacol Clin Exp 2008;23(1):1–11.

116. McElroy SL, Hudson JI, Capece JA, et al. Topiramate for the treatment of binge eating disorder associated with obesity: a placebo-controlled study. Biol Psychiatry 2007;61(9):1039–48.

117. McElroy SL, Kotwal R, Guerdjikova AI, et al. Zonisamide in the treatment of binge eating disorder with obesity: a randomized controlled trial. J Clin Psychiatry 2006;68(1):1897–906.

118. McElroy SL, Guerdjikova A, Kotwal R, et al. Atomoxetine in the treatment of binge-eating disorder: a randomized placebo-controlled trial. J Clin Psychiatry 2007;68(3):390–8.

119. Powers PS, Santana CA, Bannon YS. Olanzapine in the treatment of anorexia nervosa: an open label trial. Int J Eat Disord 2002;32(2):146–54.

120. Appolinario JC, Bacaltchuk J, Sichieri R, et al. A randomized, double-blind, placebo-controlled study of sibutramine in the treatment of binge-eating disorder. Arch Gen Psychiatry 2003;60(11):1109–16.

121. Grilo CM, Masheb RM, Salant SL. Cognitive behavioral therapy guided self-help and orlistat for the treatment of binge eating disorder: a randomized, double-blind, placebo-controlled trial. Biol Psychiatry 2005;57(10):1193–201.

122. Wilfley DE, Crow SJ, Hudson JI, et al. Efficacy of sibutramine for the treatment of binge eating disorder: a randomized multicenter placebo-controlled double-blind study. Am J Psychiatry 2008;165(1):51–8.

123. Bellini M, Merli M. Current drug treatment of patients with bulimia nervosa and binge-eating disorder: selective serotonin reuptake inhibitors versus mood stabilizers. Int J Psychiatr Clin Pract 2004;8(4):235–43.

124. Crow SJ, Mitchell JE, Roerig JD, et al. What potential role is there for medication treatment in anorexia nervosa? Int J Eat Disord 2009;42(1):1–8.

125. Pike KM, Hilbert A, Wilfley DE, et al. Toward an understanding of risk factors for anorexia nervosa: a case-control study. Psychol Med 2008;38(10):1443–53.

126. Zhu AJ, Walsh BT. Pharmacologic treatment of eating disorders. Can J Psychiatry 2002;47(3):227–34.

127. Baum A. Eating disorders in the male athlete. Sports Med 2006;36(1):1–6.

128. National Collegiate Athletic Association. 2010–11 NCAA banned drugs. PrFont34-Bin0BinSub0Frac0Def1Margin0Margin0Jc1Indent1440Lim0Lim1. Available at: http://www.ncaa.org/wps/portal/ncaahome?WCM_GLOBAL_CONTEXT=/ncaa/ncaa/legislation+and+governance/eligibility+and+recruiting/drug+testing/ncaa+banned-drug+classes. Accessed November 23, 2010.

129. Carter JC, Stewart DA, Dunn VJ, et al. Primary prevention of eating disorders: might it do more harm than good? Int J Eat Disord 1997;22(2):167–72.

130. Moreno AB, Thelen MH. A preliminary prevention program for eating disorders in a junior high school population. J Youth Adolesc 1993;22(2):109–24.

131. Stice E, Shaw H. Eating disorder prevention programs: a meta-analytic review. Psychol Bull 2004;130(2):1–23.
132. Neumark-Sztainer D, Butler R, Palti H. Eating disturbances among adolescent girls: evaluation of a school-based primary prevention program. J Nutr Educ 1995;27(1):24–31.
133. Stice E, Mazotti L, Weibel D, et al. Dissonance prevention program decreases thin-ideal internalization, body dissatisfaction, dieting, negative affect, and bulimic symptoms: a preliminary experiment. Int J Eat Disord 2000;27(2): 206–17.
134. Stoolmiller M, Eddy JM, Reid JB. Detecting and describing preventive intervention effects in a universal school-based randomized trial targeting delinquent and violent behavior. J Consult Clin Psychol 2000;68(2):296–306.
135. Elliot DL, Moe EL, Goldberg L, et al. Definition and outcome of a curriculum to prevent disordered eating and body-shaping drug use. J Sch Health 2006; 76(2):67–73.
136. Elliot DL, Goldberg L, Moe EL, et al. Long-term outcomes of the ATHENA (Athletes Targeting Healthy Exercise & Nutrition Alternatives) program for female high school athletes. J Alcohol Drug Educ 2008;52(2):73–92.
137. Stice E, Shaw H, Becker C, et al. Dissonance-based interventions for the prevention of eating disorders: using persuasion principles to promote health. Prev Sci 2008;9(2):114–28.
138. Stice E, Trost A, Chase A. Healthy weight control and dissonance-based eating disorder prevention programs: results from a controlled trial. Int J Eat Disord 2003;33(1):10–21.
139. Becker CB, Wilson C, Williams A, et al. Peer-facilitated cognitive dissonance versus healthy weight eating disorders prevention: a randomized comparison. Body Image 2010;7(4):280–8.
140. Larimer ME, Cronce JM. Identification, prevention and treatment: a review of individual-focused strategies to reduce problematic alcohol consumption by college students. J Stud Alcohol 2002;14:148–63.
141. Beck AT. Cognitive therapy: nature and relation to behavior therapy. Behav Ther 1970;1(2):184–200.
142. Telch CF, Agras WS, Linehan MM. Dialectical behavior therapy for binge eating disorder. J Consult Clin Psychol 2001;69(6):1061–5.
143. Ben-Porath DD, Wisniewski L, Warren M. Differential treatment response for eating disordered patients with and without a comorbid borderline personality diagnosis using a dialectical behavior therapy (DBT)-informed approach. Eat Disord 2009;17(3):225–41.
144. Matusek JA, Wendt SJ, Wiseman CV. Dissonance thin-ideal and didactic healthy behavior eating disorder prevention programs: results from a controlled trial. Int J Eat Disord 2004;36(4):376–88.
145. Green M, Scott N, Diyankova I, et al. Eating disorder prevention: an experimental comparison of high level dissonance, low level dissonance, and no-treatment control. Eat Disord 2005;13(2):157–69.
146. Black Becker C, Bull S, Smith LM, et al. Effects of being a peer-leader in an eating disorder prevention program: can we further reduce eating disorder risk factors? Eat Disord 2008;16(5):444–59.

Infectious Disease

Carrie A. Jaworski, MD[a,b,*], Brian Donohue, DO[c],
Joshua Kluetz, DO[c]

KEYWORDS

- Infectious disease • Infectious mononucleosis • Pertussis
- Influenza • CA-MRSA • Skin infection • Return to play

Athletes are susceptible to the same infections as the general population. However, several special considerations need to be taken into account when dealing with an athlete who has contracted an infectious disease. Health care providers need to consider how even common illnesses can affect an athlete's performance, the communicability of the illness to team members, and precautions/contraindications related to athletic participation. Recent advances in the prevention, diagnosis, and/or management of illness in general are addressed in this article. In addition, updates in certain conditions such as infectious mononucleosis, influenza, pertussis, and community-acquired methicillin-resistant *Staphylococcus aureus* skin infections warrant special attention in the athletic setting, and are discussed in detail.

IMMUNE FUNCTION AND EXERCISE

Much has been written on the proposed effects of exercise on immune function. The literature supports both the positive and negative effects that exercise can have on immune function and risk of illness.[1,2] The relationship between exercise and immune function has been described by Nieman[2] as a "J"-shaped curve. In this model, moderate exercise has been reported to enhance immune function above that of sedentary individuals while excessive, intense exercise may impair immune function. The depressive effect on immune function generally lasts 3 to 24 hours after exercise depending on intensity and duration of the activity. This effect is most pronounced when exercise is continuous, prolonged (>1.5 hours), has a 55% to 75% maximum O_2 uptake, and is performed without food intake. The immune dysfunction can last longer if this type of training lasts 1 week or more. This suppression is an obvious

[a] Intercollegiate Sports Medicine, Northwestern University, 1501 Central Street, Evanston, IL 60208, USA
[b] Department of Family and Community Medicine, Feinberg School of Medicine, Northwestern University, 710 North Lake Shore Drive, 4th Floor, Chicago, IL 60611, USA
[c] Sports Medicine Fellowship, Resurrection Medical Center, 7447 West Talcott Avenue, Chicago, IL 60631, USA
* Corresponding author. Intercollegiate Sports Medicine, Northwestern University, 1501 Central Street, Evanston, IL 60208.
E-mail address: c-jaworski@northwestern.edu

Clin Sports Med 30 (2011) 575–590
doi:10.1016/j.csm.2011.03.006
0278-5919/11/$ – see front matter © 2011 Elsevier Inc. All rights reserved.
sportsmed.theclinics.com

concern for athletes who train year-round and for whom even a minor infection can potentially hamper athletic performance. Despite this, there are very few studies that have been able to actually demonstrate a direct link between exercise-induced impaired immune function and an increased incidence of clinically confirmed infection.[1] In addition, the beneficial effects of exercise on longevity and overall health far outweigh any perceived detriment to immune function.

RESPIRATORY INFECTIONS
Upper Respiratory Tract Infection

Upper respiratory tract infections (URTI) are extremely common in both the athletic and nonathletic populations. It has been reported that a typical adult will be afflicted with a URTI 1 to 6 times per year. Most of the time symptoms will be caused by rhino-viruses, although there are several other causative agents.[3] Despite the potential protection offered by moderate exercise, respiratory infections are the most common type of infection contracted by athletes.[4,5] Infections tend to occur in early autumn through early spring, most likely due to crowding indoors and physiologic changes that occur because of the cold.[6]

Fortunately, URTIs are self-limited and the typical symptoms of rhinorrhea, sore throat, fatigue, nasal congestion, mildly elevated temperature, and cough resolve over a 7- to 10-day period. Diagnosis is generally straightforward and over-the-counter medications, including analgesics, antipyretics, and decongestants are recommended for symptom relief. Caution does need to be taken when prescribing decongestants for athletes, due to risk of dehydration and hyperthermia as well as restrictions on their use by certain sport-governing bodies. Practitioners can refer to the World Anti-Doping Agency's (WADA) Web site for the most up-to-date list of prohibited substances.[7]

Athletes with these mild viral infections can continue to compete as tolerated, as the symptoms and severity of the illness do not seem to be adversely affected by exercise.[8] Exceptions include febrile athletes, those with more severe bacterial infections such as sinusitis and pharyngitis, and those with symptoms below the neck. The "neck check" guide was first suggested by Eichner,[9] and recommends that athletes may return to sport if their symptoms are all "above the neck" (rhinorrhea, sore throat, congestion). If there are symptoms present "below the neck" (fever, malaise, gastro-intestinal symptoms), athletes should be kept from participation until symptoms have resolved.

When being treated for a bacterial infection such as sinusitis or pharyngitis, the athlete should be afebrile and on antibiotics for at least 24 hours before returning to participation. After this, a short trial of activity can be undertaken and if there is no effect on symptoms then participation may be continued. If, however, there is aggravation of significant symptoms, activity should be halted.

Infectious Mononucleosis

Infectious mononucleosis (IM) affects a significant portion of the athletic population yearly. The majority of cases occur in those between the ages of 15 and 25 years. While the typical symptoms of fever, sore throat, and lymphadenopathy are not terribly troublesome, it is the potential enlargement of the spleen that is especially concerning in this population.

The primary causative agent of IM is the Epstein-Barr virus (EBV). EBV infection is essentially ubiquitous, with more than 95% of adults worldwide being seropositive.[10] It has been estimated that anywhere from 30% to 75% of college freshmen have not had a primary EBV infection. The rate of infection is approximately 10% to 20% for this susceptible population. Of those infected, 30% to 50% will go on to develop frank IM.[11] Athletes who share water bottles, cups, and other equipment are at increased risk, as the primary mode of transmission is via oropharyngeal secretions.

Difficulty arises when attempting to contain a mononucleosis outbreak in athletic populations, due to the fact that there is a 30- to 50-day incubation period prior to symptom presentation. Commonly there will also be a 3- to 5-day prodromal course of mild flu-like symptoms. These symptoms are followed by the aforesaid classic manifestations and fatigue that is often moderate to severe. The majority of clinical findings have been found to resolve by 4 weeks, with cervical lymphadenopathy and fatigue taking a longer course.

Diagnosis of IM is based on clinical findings and laboratory data. The finding of more than 10% atypical lymphocytes has a sensitivity of 75% and a specificity of 92% for the diagnosis of IM.[12] A heterophile antibody (Monospot) test can be performed with the caveat that there is a false-negative rate of 25% in the first week and 5% to 10% during or after the second week.[13] Blood testing for EBV-specific IgG and IgM antibodies should be performed for definitive diagnosis. The presence of IgM signifies an acute EBV infection, while IgG levels increase several weeks later and remain elevated for life.

The most frequent complication of IM is concomitant group A *Streptococcus* pharyngitis, which has been reported to occur in up to 30% of cases.[14] It has been proposed that screening with rapid antigen test or culture for group A strepotococcal (GAS) infection should be considered in light of the high coinfection rate and potential sequelae of untreated strep pharyngitis.[10] Penicillin continues to be the drug of choice, and can be given either as a one-time intramuscular dose or by oral route for 10 days. Erythromycin is an alternative in those who are allergic to penicillin. Amoxicillin should not be used for GAS in the face of concomitant IM, as a nonallergic rash will result 80% to 90% of the time.[15]

Oral steroids have a role in the treatment of complications arising from IM, including tonsillar hypertrophy and some hematologic abnormalities. Their use has been proposed as a primary treatment of IM, but the data does not show a clinically relevant benefit.[16] The use of antivirals such as acyclovir or valacyclovir for acute IM has also been proposed. Limited research in this area has not supported their routine use.[10]

A widely feared complication is splenic rupture. Splenic rupture is a rare complication occurring in only 0.1% to 0.2% of those with IM.[17] Splenomegaly is thought to occur in 50% to 100% of IM cases as a result of lymphocytic infiltration that distorts the support structure of the spleen, leading to fragility. The majority of reported cases of splenic rupture are nontraumatic, and occur between 3 and 7 weeks after diagnosis. However, the great concern with athletes is that premature return to sport may put them at increased risk for trauma-induced splenic rupture. Unfortunately, there are no evidence-based guidelines to follow when determining return to sport. Recent research has focused on using ultrasonography as a way to guide decision making. Hosey and colleagues[18] performed ultrasonography of the spleen on a large cohort of healthy college athletes and found that there was a wide range of spleen sizes. Spleen size correlated with height and weight but not with sex or race. Another group looked at tall athletes, and found that spleen size is larger in taller athletes than in the average individual.[19]

A subsequent study[20] performing serial ultrasound measurements on athletes with IM was performed, and has helped to further establish current recommendations for return to play. Healthy athletes had splenic ultrasonography performed as a baseline. Those who went on to develop IM had serial ultrasound scans. Data were obtained from 20 such athletes over a 5-year period. It was found that peak splenic enlargement was reached within 2 weeks from symptom onset, but could take as long as 3.5 weeks. Following peak enlargement, the spleen decreased in size by approximately 1% per day.[20] The results support the general recommendation that athletes should be held from physical activity for 3 weeks from onset of symptoms before returning to light activity. However, it should be noted that a direct relationship between the size of the spleen and risk of rupture in individuals with IM has not been established.[21]

Based on the aforementioned data, it becomes apparent that the question of when it is safe to allow an athlete with IM to return to play is difficult for the clinician to answer. Expert recommendations continue to guide this complex decision. It is generally well accepted that once the athlete is afebrile and appropriately hydrated, fatigue has improved, and a minimum period of 3 weeks has passed from symptom onset, he or she may be allowed to slowly return to light, noncontact activities. If the athlete does not experience any worsening of symptoms, he or she may be allowed to progress to more strenuous activity and finally to full participation.[21–23] Return to play should be individualized and sound clinical judgment used.

Bronchitis and Pertussis

Cough that lasts for more than 10 days but less than 3 weeks and is of infectious origin is referred to as acute bronchitis. Viruses are the causative agents 90% of the time. It is rare that testing is needed to confirm the diagnosis. Therapy is directed at symptom relief for the majority of bronchitis cases. Evidence does not support the routine use of antibiotics.[24] Many patients, especially athletes, expect antibiotics as a "quick fix," and it is important to explain the reasoning as to why it should not be done (ie, antibiotic resistance, *Clostridium difficile* infection, and so forth). Some have suggested that antibiotics be prescribed to prevent subsequent pneumonia. This idea is not supported in the literature. It has been found that 119 patients in the 16- to 64-year-old population with acute bronchitis would need to be treated with antibiotics to prevent one case of pneumonia.[25]

When cough lasts beyond 3 weeks, alternative diagnoses should be considered. Common causes include asthma, postnasal drip, gastroesophageal reflux, and infection with *Bordetella pertussis*. Since the development of a vaccine against pertussis, the associated morbidity and mortality has significantly decreased. Infection in adults is usually mild and self-limited, but this group may act as a reservoir for infants and unvaccinated children who bear the brunt of poor outcomes.[26] In addition, a prolonged cough in an athlete can be a significant detriment to their performance. Since the 1980s, there has been an increase in pertussis cases among teens and, as such, the Advisory Council on Immunization Practices (ACIP) has recommended a booster vaccine for adolescents and adults as immunity from childhood vaccination decreases after 5 to 10 years.[27,28] As of 2010, ACIP approved the use of tetanus/diphtheria/acellular pertussis (Tdap) regardless of one's last tetanus-toxoid or diphtheria-toxoid containing vaccine, in an attempt to curtail pertussis in the United States. ACIP recommends a single Tdap dose for persons aged 11 to 18 years who have completed the primary series and for adults aged 19 to 64 years.[29] In the athletic setting, providers should educate their athletes and staff about the need for such vaccination.

Unfortunately, there is little to help the clinician distinguish pertussis from other causes of chronic cough. A review of the data in 2010 found paroxysmal cough to be the most common finding; however, this finding lacked specificity. The classic symptoms of posttussive emesis and "whoop" are not commonly seen in clinical practice. Their presence does increase the specificity of pertussis, but the presence or absence of these classic symptoms is not enough to definitively diagnose or rule out pertussis.[30] Laboratory testing for pertussis begins by obtaining a nasopharyngeal specimen that can be sent for either culture or a polymerase chain reaction (PCR). Sensitivity and specificity of culture are poor, and results take several days to obtain. PCR is much quicker, with results available in 1 to 2 days, but it is costly. Because of the limitations of the currently available tests, most suspected cases are treated based on recent exposures and patient presentation.[30]

Regimes for treatment and postexposure prophylaxis are identical. In confirmed cases of pertussis, teammates should be considered for chemoprophylaxis. Macrolides continue to be the antibiotic of choice with the use of trimethoprim-sulfamethoxazole (TMP-SMX) when macrolides cannot be used. For athletes with confirmed pertussis on therapy, it is recommended by the American College of Chest Physicians (ACCP) that they be isolated for the first 5 days of antibiotic treatment.[24,31]

Influenza

Influenza is a highly contagious viral respiratory illness that is best prevented through vaccination and strict respiratory hygiene. The virus is spread quickly and easily via respiratory droplets, especially in places where there is crowding and poor hygiene.

Athletes are at increased risk based on their close proximity to others during practice, games, and travel.

Influenza activity peaks during the winter months. Historically, influenza A and B have a greater impact on the unhealthy, the very young, and the elderly. The recent H1N1 pandemic of 2009 highlighted the challenges a health care system faces in the absence of an available vaccine. In 2009–2010, H1N1 influenza A resulted in approximately 400,000 hospitalizations compared with the 200,000 seen in a normal flu season.[32] Those younger than 18 years proved to be particularly susceptible.[33] Strong educational initiatives on hand washing, adherence to Centers for Disease Control and Prevention (CDC) isolation guidelines, and the early reporting of symptoms helped to curtail many H1N1 outbreaks at the high school, collegiate, and professional sports levels.

Typically a patient with influenza will present with fever, dry cough, headache, and myalgias. Sore throat, rhinorrhea, and congestion are other common physical findings. Influenza is the most common cause of viral pneumonia. When pneumonia is suspected a chest radiograph should be obtained, as the presence of an infiltrate is required for diagnosis.

The diagnosis of influenza is usually clinical, as confirmation of infection with laboratory testing does not typically change the management. If desired, or the diagnosis is in doubt, nasal washings or a pharyngeal swab may be obtained. The vast majority of otherwise healthy individuals infected with influenza will go on to complete resolution with only symptomatic treatment.[34] Symptom improvement occurs between days 3 and 7, with cough and fatigue lasting days longer.

Antiviral treatment against influenza A and B is available in the form of neuraminidase inhibitors (oseltamivir and zanamivir). For maximum effectiveness, this class of medication needs to be started within 48 hours of symptom onset. In the otherwise healthy outpatient population, these medications only have mild to moderate effect.[35] Resistance is variable and changes over time. There was near universal resistance of H1N1 to oseltamivir, with good susceptibility to zanamivir during the 2009 pandemic.[36] Neuraminidase inhibitors can be considered for chemoprophylaxis in high-risk household contacts. In the 2009 outbreak, athletes were not considered high-risk contacts and did not qualify for chemoprophylaxis based on CDC guidelines, mainly due to a fear of antiviral shortages during the pandemic.

Prevention with vaccination is the most important management strategy. Previously only certain groups had been the focus of vaccination efforts. As of this writing, ACIP recommends universal vaccination for those older than 6 months.[37] In-season athletes should be highly encouraged to obtain an influenza vaccine.

GASTROINTESTINAL
Traveler's Diarrhea

Traveler's diarrhea (TD) is a common illness that affects many travelers, including athletes. Many athletes travel outside of their local communities and compete at the national and international level. TD is usually a self-limited disease process; however, the resultant dehydration can adversely affect an athlete's performance. The classic presentation of TD includes 3 or more unformed stools in 24 hours, nausea, vomiting, fever, abdominal cramping, or bloody stools. Most cases last between 1 and 5 days and occur within the first 4 to 14 days of travel.[38]

Acute TD can be divided into bacterial, viral, or parasitic varieties. About 90% of cases are bacterial, with a majority of those being caused by *Escherichia coli*.[39] Other bacteria to consider include *Salmonella* species, *Shigella* species, *Vibrio* species, and *Campylobacter* species. Viral causes make up 5% to 10% of TD cases, with the most frequent causative organism being Norovirus. These viruses are all transmitted via the fecal-oral route. Though accounting for a small percentage of TD cases, parasitic infections should be considered in athletes who have persistent symptoms (longer than 7 days).The common parasites include *Giardia lamblia*, *Cryptosporidium parvum*, and *Cyclospora cayetanensis*.

Diagnosis of TD is usually made by clinical presentation without the causative organism being identified, due to its generally benign and self-limited course. However, if the TD lasts greater than 7 days or the patient has fever or colitis symptoms (fever, tenesmus, urgency, cramping, or bloody diarrhea), stool cultures should be done.[40,41]

The first line of treatment for TD is fluid replacement. Antibiotic therapy should be considered in athletes who develop severe diarrhea, classified as greater than 4 unformed stools a day, fever, blood, pus, or mucus in the stool. Flouroquinolones have typically been the drug of choice for TD. However, the rare risk of tendon rupture in a young athlete may warrant consideration of an alternative antibiotic choice. Azithromycin has been shown to be equally as effective for TD as flouroquinolones.[42] Ciprofloxacin is dosed at 500 mg twice daily for 1 to 2 days or azithromycin is given as a 1000 mg single dose. In TD caused by *E coli*, rifaximin has effectiveness that is equivalent to the flouroquinolones.[43] For other types of TD that cause fever or bloody stools, such as *Campylobacter*, rifaximin is not effective.[43] If the TD is suspected to be caused by parasitic infection, metronidazole, 500 mg 3 times daily for 5 days is an appropriate empiric regimen.

The use of antimotility agents such as loperamide and diphenoxylate has been controversial in the past; however, recently these therapies have been considered safe when taken with an antibiotic. More conservative recommendations for athletes suggest only using them sparingly, such as during a competition or lengthy travel.[44]

GENITOURINARY
Urinary Tract Infections

Urinary tract infection (UTI) is an exceedingly common diagnosis that affects women disproportionately more than men. It is reported that before age 24 years, one-third of all women will have experienced at least one UTI. In the second and third decades of life, women are 35 times more likely than their male counterparts to be stricken with a UTI.[45] Based on these numbers it is clear that suspected UTI is a common reason for female high school and college athletes to seek medical attention.

The most common pathogen in both sexes is *E coli*, accounting for nearly 85% of cases in females. Antibiotic treatment options are well established, and the ultimate decision is often based on patient allergies and local rates of resistance. Of note, the often prescribed antibiotic TMP-SMX has seen a large increase in the rate of resistance in the past 20 years.[46] Resistance rates vary based on location, but it is still considered an appropriate initial choice when rates are below 20%.[47] A short, 3-day course of treatment is favored for females with uncomplicated infection.[48] In addition to requiring both urinalysis and urine culture for workup of cystitis, men require a longer 7-day course of therapy.[49]

A few small studies have suggested that drinking cranberry juice may decrease the incidence of UTIs. A recent placebo-controlled trial involving college-aged women with previous UTI found that the recurrence rate neared 20% in the cranberry juice arm and only 14% in the placebo arm.[50] Further investigation is warranted.

Sexually Transmitted Infections

Sexually transmitted infections (STIs) continue to have a major impact on society. Men and women younger than 25 years bear the greatest burden, with minority populations having the highest rates. As many athletes fall within this age range, educational initiatives are paramount in preventing spread of disease. Recent published data by the CDC reports "approximately 19 million new STIs per year, which cost the U.S. healthcare system $16.4 billion annually."[51]

The 3 STIs most likely to be seen in a young athletic population are *Chlamydia*, gonorrhea, and human papillomavirus (HPV). All 3 warrant screening and education on prevention. Gardasil is a 3-dose HPV vaccine recommended for females between the ages of 9 and 26 years. Although it does not protect against all strains, it offers protection against several of the strains most highly associated with cervical cancer. The CDC maintains a comprehensive database of up-to-date diagnosis and treatment guidelines for all STIs on their Web site.[51]

Return-to-play guidelines depend on the cause of infection. Uncomplicated chlamydial or gonorrheal urethritis/cervicitis/rectal disease will rarely preclude participation. If complications develop, such as epididymitis, pelvic inflammatory disease, or disseminated gonorrheal disease, the athlete should be held from competition until aggressively treated and all symptoms have resolved.[23]

Blood-Borne Infections

Hepatitis B virus (HBV) is transmitted parenterally, by sexual intercourse, perinatally, and to a much lesser degree by mucosal contact with infected blood or bodily secretions. The incubation period is 45 to 160 days, and most patients recover spontaneously. However, 6% to 10% of patients will progress to chronic infection.[40] It is believed that HBV is 100 times more transmissible than human immunodeficiency virus (HIV) and 10 times more transmissible than hepatitis C.[52] Prevention of HBV infection includes vaccination for all children as well as those adults who have a higher risk due to their occupation or lifestyle. Standard precautions should be used when treating athletes who may have open wounds or are bleeding because of injury. The position of the National Collegiate Athletic Association (NCAA) on athletes with HBV infection is that they should be allowed to participate in sports as long as they do not have an acute infection or have symptoms of systemic disease. Although the risk of transmission is limited in the athletic setting, the risk is higher in HBV than in hepatitis C virus (HCV) or HIV. The NCAA guideline states that if the athlete has an acute HBV infection, it is prudent to remove the athlete from close-contact sports, such as wrestling, until loss of infectivity is proven as determined by absence of the HBV e antigen (HBeAg). Athletes with chronic HBV infections who are HBeAg positive should probably be removed from competition indefinitely because they are at the highest risk of transmitting HBV.[53]

HCV is transmitted through contact with blood or blood products, injecting drugs, or needle-stick exposures. Incubation is 14 to 180 days, and seroprevalence of HCV in the United States is 1.8%.[54] The major concern with HCV infection is that up to 70% of patients develop chronic infection, of which about one-quarter will progress to frank cirrhosis.[40] There have been no reported cases of HCV acquisition during sports-related activities. Off-the-field behaviors likely have a higher risk of HCV transmission, such as the use of injectable steroids and other performance enhancers.[55]

HUMAN IMMUNODEFICIENCY VIRUS

About 1 million Americans are infected with HIV. Although there is no cure for HIV, medical treatment has enabled patients to achieve very low viral load counts and to lead very active and productive lives. When compared with HBV, HIV is less stable and also has less infectivity.[52,53] HIV is much more likely to be transmitted via exposure to blood or needle-stick exposure than through athletic competition. There have been no confirmed cases of HIV transmission in sports, and the risk of an athlete acquiring HIV appears to be greatest from high-risk behaviors conducted off the field.[40,56]

Because there is no cure or vaccine for HIV, prevention is the key to prevent the spread of HIV in athletics. Universal precautions should always be used when caring for athletes. These precautions comprise proper wound care including appropriate dressings, making the equipment and materials comply with standard precautions readily available, maintaining vigilance in wound surveillance, and the appropriate cleaning of contaminated equipment and uniforms.[40,53,56]

SKIN AND SOFT TISSUE INFECTIONS

Due to the nature of most sports, athletes are in constant contact with other athletes and with potentially contaminated surfaces, and/or experience skin breakdown, all of which lead to an increased risk of skin infection. Once an athlete sustains a skin infection, the goal of the sports medicine provider is to not only treat the infection but to also prevent spread of the infection to other participants. The National Athletic Trainers Association (NATA), the NCAA, and the National Federation of State High School Associations (NFSH) have established return-to-play guidelines for common skin infections, which are outlined in **Table 1**.[53,57,58]

Tineas

These superficial cutaneous infections are caused by the dermatophytes *Trychophyton rubrum*, *Trychophyton tonsurans*, *Microsporum* sp, and *Epidermophyton floccusum*. These infections infect many areas of the body, and are named by area. Dermatophyte infection of the scalp is tinea capitis. Infections on the body are named tinea corporis, commonly called ringworm, and infections in the groin are called tinea cruris, or jock-itch. Lastly, infections of the feet are known as tinea pedis and of the toenails, onychomycosis.[59]

Diagnosis of tinea can often be made clinically. Direct microscopy of scrapings from the border of the lesion can be performed after it is prepared with potassium hydroxide (KOH) if the diagnosis is uncertain. If the diagnosis is still in question, the most definitive test is a fungal culture.[57,59]

Table 1
Return-to-play guidelines for common skin infections

	Tinea	Herpes Simplex	Molluscum	Impetigo
NCAA/NATA	Capitis: Oral fungicidal agent × 2 wk Corporis: Topical fungicidal for minimum of 72 h. Cover with gas-permeable membrane Pedis: No rules	Primary: Oral antivirals for 120 h, no new lesions or systemic symptoms for 72 h Recurrent: 120 h of oral antivirals and no new moist lesions	Solitary lesions: Cover with gas-permeable membrane Numerous: Curette or remove	72 h of topical or oral antibiotic therapy, no new lesions for 72 h, and lesions covered to contain drainage Same for other staphylococcal or streptococcal skin infections such as furuncles, cellulitis, etc
NFHS	Capitis: Same as above Corporis: 7 days of oral or topical fungicidal and written release from physician or coach Pedis: No rules	Same as NCAA	Same as NCAA	Oral antibiotics for at least 48 h, no draining or moist lesions

Abbreviations: NATA, National Athletic Trainers Association; NCAA, National Collegiate Athletic Association; NFHS, National Federation of High School Associations.
Data from Refs.[53,57,58]

Treatment of these superficial cutaneous fungal infections will vary depending on location. Tinea capitis must be treated with an oral agent, whereas tinea corporis and tinea cruris can be treated with topical therapy initially. The topical agents are well tolerated, with the oral agents having a higher risk for side effects. The chosen therapies should be fungicidal for the best outcome.

For a majority of cases, topical terbinafine 1% cream can be applied once to twice daily for 2 to 4 weeks or ketoconazole 2% cream can be applied once daily for 2 to 4 weeks. For patients who fail topical therapy, oral regimens can be used. Griseofulvin can be prescribed at 500 mg daily for 2 to 4 weeks, while monitoring for adverse side effects including paresthesias, elevated serum transaminases, headache, and photosensitivity. Other options include terbinafine 250 mg daily for 1 week, itraconazole 100 mg daily for 2 weeks, or fluconazole 150 mg once a week for 2 to 4 weeks.[60]

Prophylactic use of fluconazole has been used to reduce the incidence of tinea in wrestlers. Brickman and colleagues[61] report that by using fluconazole 100 mg daily for 3 days at 2 points during the wrestling season, the incidence of tinea gladiatorum decreased from 67.4% to 3.5%. The wrestlers also had no adverse side effects from this regimen during the 10-year study period.

Herpes Simplex (Herpes Gladiatorum)

Herpes simplex virus (HSV) type 1 that occurs in relation to sports participation is referred to as herpes gladiatorum, due to its high prevalence in wrestlers. This type of HSV is transmitted via skin-to-skin contact and occurs predominately on the head, face, and neck. The incubation time, or time from initial exposure to vesicle eruption, has been found to be 6.8 to 1.7 days. The likelihood of contracting herpes from an infected training partner with an active outbreak was found to be 32%.[62]

Clinical presentation of a primary HSV infection can start with mild flu-like symptoms followed by eruptions of vesicles on an erythematous base 1 to 2 days later. Flu-like symptoms can include fever, malaise, pharyngitis, lymphadenopathy, and conjunctivitis. Subsequent infections will usually have less systemic symptoms.

HSV infection can be diagnosed on clinical presentation or Tzanck preparations of fluid from an unroofed vesicle. Viral cultures can also be done but require several days for results.[59]

Treatment of herpes gladiatorum includes acyclovir at different dosing regimens for primary versus recurrent infection. Valacyclovir offers an easier dosing regimen if compliance is a concern.[63]

The prevention of herpes gladiatorum should include personal hygiene, cleaning of shared equipment, and daily skin checks. Suppressive therapy with antiviral medications such as acyclovir and valacyclovir is also an option. Recommended regimens used for suppression include acyclovir 400 mg twice daily, valacyclovir 500 to 1000 mg daily, or famcyclovir 250 mg twice daily.[63] Some research has recommended conducting annual HSV serologic testing and placing HSV-seropositive athletes on suppressive therapy at the beginning of every season. Those athletes who are HSV-seronegative should be tested annually to detect seroconversion.[64]

Molluscum Contagiosum

Molluscum contagiosum is a viral skin infection that is commonly seen in athletes. This viral infection is transmitted via direct skin-to-skin contact with an infected individual. The classic lesions are commonly located on the trunk and face, and appear as round, flesh-colored papules with an umbilicated center. Smaller lesions may not have an umbilicated center and may be confused with the common wart.[40]

In healthy individuals, this infection is usually self-limited and lasts about 6 months without treatment. Faster treatment is usually desired in the athletic setting, thus surgical and nonsurgical options are available. Curettage or cryotherapy are common treatment options and offer the fastest treatment. Chemical destruction with 0.7% cantharidin solution is also a widely used treatment. Self-administered treatment for several weeks with topical imiquimod or phyllotoxin has been studied and has been shown to be an effective treatment for molluscum contagiosum.[65,66]

Impetigo

One of the most common skin infections found in athletes, impetigo is a superficial skin infection caused by *Staphylococcus* or *Streptococcus* species, or a combination of the two. Transmission is by direct skin-to-skin contact with an infected athlete, and can be found on both broken and unbroken skin. These lesions are typically covered in a honey-colored crust. Postinfectious complications are rare, but the most significant is pyelonephritis in association with some strains.[40,67]

For limited infections, topical mupirocin applied twice daily for 10 days can be used. If the impetigo is diffuse, systemic antibiotics can be used together with topical therapy. Common regimens include cephalexin 500 mg 3 to 4 times daily for 10 days or dicloxacillin 500 mg 3 to 4 times daily for 10 days.

Folliculitis, Furunculosis, and Cellulitis

Infection of the hair follicle is commonly caused by *Staphylococcus* and *Streptococcus* species. Infections of the upper part of the follicle are classified as folliculitis, and deeper infections of the lower follicle are classified as furuncles. These infections are spread by direct skin-to-skin contact. Folliculitis presents as small, tender lesions on an erythematous base, and is usually located in areas that are occluded by athletic equipment. On the other hand, furuncles are typically larger, tender, and appear as firm pustules or abscesses. Furuncles are often surrounded by an area of cellulitis.[40] Cellulitis is a skin infection that includes the dermis and the subcutaneous tissues, and is characterized by erythema, edema, and pain. The most common infectious agents include group A streptococcus and *Staphylococcus aureus*. Local trauma, abrasions, or any other disruption of the skin can increase the risk of cellulitis.

Diagnosis of folliculitis and furunculosis is typically made by clinical appearance. However, in light of the increasing frequency of community-acquired methicillin-resistant *S aureus* (CA-MRSA) cases, furuncles and abscesses should be incised and cultured.[40,67]

Treatment of localized folliculitis can be accomplished with topical mupirocin. If the infection is more diffuse, oral antibiotics should be used. Antibiotic decisions should be based on the extent of the infection and the prevalence of MRSA in the community. Less severe infections can be treated with cephalexin 500 mg 4 times daily for 7 to 10 days, with close follow-up to monitor treatment response. Extensive cellulitis, or lesions worsening on oral antibiotics, may require hospitalization for intravenous antibiotics.[67]

COMMUNITY-ACQUIRED METHICILLIN-RESISTANT *STAPHYLOCOCCUS AUREUS*

Over the last 20 years the emergence of MRSA has changed the way skin infections are treated. CA-MRSA can manifest in otherwise young and healthy patients, often including athletes. Established risk factors for CA-MRSA infections comprise poor hygiene, overcrowded living conditions, direct skin-to-skin contact, sharing contaminated personal items, and trauma to the skin. Outbreaks of MRSA skin infections have occurred in athletes involved in contact sports such as wrestling, football, rugby, and fencing. Infection often occurs at turf-abrasion sites or other areas of injured skin, and in athletes who share equipment.[68] One recent study demonstrated that nasal colonization rates of MRSA in collegiate athletes fluctuated, showing the highest rates during the peak of the athletic season. For a men's football team, colonization rates ranged from 12% to 30% and for a women's lacrosse team, the rate ranged from 28% to 39%.[69]

Skin and soft tissue infections caused by CA-MRSA clinically present as an abscess or necrotic-appearing lesion. These lesions can be accompanied by fever, surrounding cellulitis, or even bacteremia. Clinicians should not rely on appearance alone, and thus the diagnosis should be confirmed by wound culture. For an abscess less than 5 cm in size, incision and drainage is often adequate treatment. However, because of the location of the infection and reliability of the patient, concomitant use of oral antibiotics is usually recommended. Due to the prevalence of CA-MRSA, empiric oral antibiotic regimens should include coverage for both methicillin-sensitive *S aureus* and MRSA. Appropriate first-line agents include TMP-SMX DS twice daily or doxycycline 100 mg twice daily for 10 to 14 days. Second-line agents such as clindamycin 300 mg 4 times daily or linezolid 600 mg twice daily for 10 to 14 days should be used with caution, due to high levels of inducible resistance.[70,71] Severe infections with systemic symptoms such as fever, or in patients with other comorbid medical diagnoses, may need inpatient intravenous antibiotic therapy.

For patients with recurrent MRSA infections, it is reasonable to perform a nasal culture to determine if they are colonized. However, the effectiveness of decolonization therapy is limited. A double-blind, placebo-controlled 5-day trial of topical mupirocin placed in the anterior nares together with chlorhexidine soap for the skin was successful in only 25% of patients in the mupirocin group compared with an even poorer 18% in the group using chlorhexidine alone. Low-level mupirocin resistance was associated with treatment failure.[72] A recent study conducted on a professional football team challenges the utility of performing routine colonization screening. Initial nasal cultures for CA-MRSA were negative for all 108 subjects at the start of the season. During the study period, 5 players developed CA-MRSA skin infections yet were all still negative for CA-MRSA colonization at the time of the infection.[53,73,74]

Athletes with CA-MRSA skin infections can return to play once on appropriate antibiotic therapy for 72 hours and with no new lesions for 48 hours, as per NCAA guidelines. The NFHS requires 48 hours of therapy before an athlete can return to play.[53,58]

SUMMARY

A good working knowledge of the common infectious diseases that can be encountered by an athlete as well as the caveats in their management is essential in the comprehensive care of athletes. Many resources exist to aid the health care provider in providing the most up-to-date treatment that will allow for the safest and most prudently rapid return to play.

REFERENCES

1. Gleeson M. Immune function in sport and exercise. J Appl Physiol 2007;103: 693–9.
2. Nieman DC. Exercise, infection and immunity. Int J Sports Med 1994;15:S131–41.
3. Beneson AS. Acute viral respiratory diseases in control of communicable diseases in man. Washington, DC: American Public Health Association; 1975. p. 262–6.
4. Orhant E, Carling C, Cox A. A three-year prospective study of illness in professional soccer players. Res Sports Med 2010;18(3):199–204.
5. Mountjoy M, Junge A, Alonso JM, et al. Sports injuries and illnesses in the 2009 FINA World Championships (Aquatics). Br J Sports Med 2010;44(7):522–7.
6. Castellani JW, Brenner IK, Rhind SG. Cold exposure: human immune responses and intracellular cytokine expression. Med Sci Sports Exerc 2002;34:2013–20.
7. WADA Prohibited List. Available at: http://www.wada-ama.org/en/World-Anti-Doping-Program/Sports-and-Anti-Doping-Organizations/International-Standards/Prohibited-List/. Accessed January 3, 2011.
8. Metz JP. Upper respiratory tract infections: who plays, who sits? Curr Sports Med Rep 2003;2:84–90.
9. Eichner ER. Infection, immunity, and exercise: what to tell your patients. Phys Sportsmed 1993;21:125.
10. Luzuriaga K, Sullivan JL. Infectious mononucleosis. N Engl J Med 2010;362: 1993–9.
11. Crawford DH, Macsween KF, Higgins CD, et al. A cohort study among university students: identification of risk factors for Epstein-Barr virus seroconversion and infectious mononucleosis. Clin Infect Dis 2006;43:276–82.
12. Ebell MH. Epstein-Barr virus infectious mononucleosis. Am Fam Physician 2004; 70:1279–87.

13. Vidrih JA, Walensky RP, Sax PE, et al. Positive Epstein-Barr virus heterophile antibody tests in patients with primary human immunodeficiency virus infection. Am J Med 2001;111:192–4.
14. Kinderknecht JJ. Infectious mononucleosis and the spleen. Curr Sports Med Rep 2002;1:116–20.
15. Bennett NJ, Domachowske J. Mononucleosis and Epstein-Barr virus infection. Available at: http://emedicine.medscape.com/article/963894-overview. Accessed January 4, 2011.
16. Candy B, Hotopf M. Steroids for symptom control in infectious mononucleosis. Cochrane Database Syst Rev 2006;3:CD004402.
17. Farley DR, Zietlow SP, Bannon MP, et al. Spontaneous rupture of the spleen due to infectious mononucleosis. Mayo Clin Proc 1992;67:846–53.
18. Hosey RG, Mattacola CG, Kriss V, et al. Ultrasound assessment of spleen size in collegiate athletes. Br J Sports Med 2006;40:251–4.
19. McCorkle R, Thomas B, Suffaletto H, et al. Normative spleen size in tall healthy athletes: Implications for safe return to contact sports after infectious mononucleosis. Clin J Sport Med 2010;20:413–5.
20. Hosey RG, Kriss V, Uhl TL, et al. Ultrasonographic evaluation of splenic enlargement in athletes with acute infectious mononucleosis. Br J Sports Med 2008;42:974–7.
21. Putukian M, O'Connor FG, Stricker P, et al. Mononucleosis and athletic participation: an evidence-based subject review. Clin J Sport Med 2008;18:309–15.
22. Waninger KN, Harcke HT. Determination of safe return to play for athletes recovering from infectious mononucleosis. Clin J Sport Med 2005;15:410–6.
23. Hosey RG, Rodenberg RE. Infectious disease and the collegiate athlete. Clin Sports Med 2007;26:449–71.
24. Braman SS. Chronic cough due to acute bronchitis: ACCP evidence-based clinical practice guidelines. Chest 2006;129(Suppl 1):955–1035.
25. Petersen I, Johnson AM, Islam A, et al. Protective effect of antibiotics against serious complications of common respiratory tract infections: retrospective cohort study with the UK General Practice Research Database. BMJ 2007;335:982.
26. Edwards KM. Overview of pertussis: focus on epidemiology, sources of infection, and long term protection after infant vaccination. Pediatr Infect Dis J 2005;24: S104–8.
27. Kr Broder, Cortese MM, Iskander JK, et al. Advisory Committee on Immunization Practices. Preventing tetanus, diphtheria, and pertussis among adolescents: use of tetanus toxoid, reduced diphtheria toxoid and acellular pertussis vaccines recommendations of the Advisory Committee on Immunization Practices (ACIP). MMWR Recomm Rep 2006;55:1–34.
28. Kretsinger K, Kr Broder, Cortese MM, et al. Centers for Disease Control and Prevention; Advisory Committee on Immunization Practices: Healthcare Infection Control Practices Advisory Committee. Preventing tetanus, diphtheria, and pertussis among adults: use of tetanus toxoid, reduced diphtheria toxoid and acellular pertussis vaccine recommendations of the ACIP. MMWR Recomm Rep 2006;55:1–37.
29. Centers for Disease Control and Prevention. Pertussis: summary of vaccine recommendations. Available at: http://www.cdc.gov/vaccines/vpd-vac/pertussis/recs-summary.htm. Accessed January 4, 2011.
30. Cornia PB, Hersh AL, Lipshy BA, et al. Does this coughing adolescent or adult patient have pertussis? JAMA 2010;304:890–6.
31. Centers for Disease Control and Prevention. Guidelines for pertussis. Available at: http://www.CDC.gov/vaccines/pubs/pertussis-guide/downloads/chapter8.pdf. Accessed December 14, 2010.

32. Centers for Disease Control and Prevention. Updated CDC estimates of 2009 H1N1 influenza cases, hospitalizations and deaths in the United States, April 2009-April 10, 2010. Available at: http://www.cdc.gov/h1n1flu/estimates_2009_h1n1.htm. Accessed December 14, 2010.

33. Dawood FS, Jain S, Finelli L, et al. Novel Swine-Origin Influenza A (H1N1) Virus Investigation Team. Emergence of a novel swine-origin influenza A (H1N1) virus in humans. N Engl J Med 2009;360:2605–15.

34. Treanor JJ, Hayden FG, Vrooman PS, et al. US Oral Neuraminidase Study Group. Efficacy and safety of the oral neuraminidase inhibitor oseltamivir in treating acute influenza: a randomized controlled trial. JAMA 2000;283:1016–24.

35. Jefferson T, Jones M, Doshi P, et al. Neuraminidase inhibitors for preventing and treating influenza in healthy adults: systemic review and meta-analysis. BMJ 2009;339:b5106.

36. Harper SA, Bradley JS, Englund JA, et al. Seasonal influenza in adults and children-diagnosis, treatment, chemoprophylaxis, and institutional outbreak management: clinical practice guidelines of the Infectious Diseases Society of America. Clin Infect Dis 2009;48:1003–32.

37. Advisory Committee on Immunization Practices. ACIP provisional recommendations for the use of influenza vaccines. Available at: http://www.cdc.gov/flu/professionals/acip/flu_vax1011.htm#box1. Accessed December 14, 2010.

38. Hill DR. Occurrence and self-treatment of diarrhea in a large cohort of Americans traveling to developing countries. Am J Trop Med Hyg 2000;62:585–9.

39. DuPont HL, Ericsson CD. Prevention and treatment of travelers' diarrhea. N Engl J Med 1990;328:1821–7.

40. DeLee JC, Drez D, Miller MD. DeLee and Drez's Orthopaedic Sports Medicine. 3rd edition. Philadelphia: WB Saunders; 2009. Chapter 3.

41. Goodgame R. Emerging causes of traveler's diarrhea: Cryptosporidium, Cyclospora, Isospora, and Microsporidia. Curr Infect Dis Rep 2003;5:66–73.

42. Adachi JA, Ericsson CD, Jiang ZD, et al. Azithromycin found to be comparable to levofloxacin for the treatment of US travelers with acute diarrhea acquired in Mexico. Clin Infect Dis 2003;37:1165–71.

43. Adachi JA, DuPont HL. Rifaximin: a novel nonabsorbed refamycin for gastrointestinal disorders. Clin Infect Dis 2006;42:541–7.

44. Murphy GS, Bodhidatta L, Echeverria P, et al. Ciprofloxacin and loperamide in the treatment of bacillary dysentery. Ann Intern Med 1993;118:582–6.

45. Dielubanza EJ, Schaeffer AJ. Urinary tract infections in women. Med Clin North Am 2011;95:27–41.

46. Zhanel GG, Hisanaga TL, Laing NM, et al. Antibiotic resistance in outpatient urinary isolates: final results from the North American urinary tract infection collaborative alliance (NAUTICA). Int J Antimicrob Agents 2006;27:468–75.

47. Wagenlehner FM, Weidner W, Naber KG. An update on uncomplicated urinary tract infections in women. Curr Opin Urol 2009;19:268–74.

48. Milo G, Katchman E, Paul M, et al. Duration of antibacterial treatment for uncomplicated urinary tract infections in women. Cochrane Database Syst Rev 2005;2:CD004682.

49. Raynor MC, Carson CC III. Urinary infections in men. Med Clin North Am 2011;95:43–54.

50. Barbosa-Cesnik C, Brown MB, Buxton M, et al. Cranberry juice fails to prevent recurrent urinary tract infection: results from a randomized placebo-controlled trial. Clin Infect Dis 2011;52:23–30.

51. Centers for Disease Control and Prevention. Trends in sexually transmitted diseases in the United States: 2009 national data for gonorrhea, chlamydia and

syphilis. 2010. Available at: http://www.cdc.gov/std/stats09/trends.htm. Accessed December 14, 2010.

52. Pope HG Jr, Katz DL, Champoux R. Anabolic-androgenic steroid use among 1,010 college men. Phys Sportsmed 1988;16:75–84.

53. NCAA 2010-11 Sports Medicine Handbook. Guideline 21-Blood-borne Pathogens and Intercollegiate Athletics. Indianapolis (IN): NCAA; p. 66–71.

54. American Academy of Pediatrics Committee on Infectious Deisease. Hepatitis C virus infection. Elk Grove Village (IL): American Academy of Pediatrics; 1998.

55. Gutierrez RL, Decker CF. Blood-borne infections and the athlete. Dis Mon 2010; 56:436–42.

56. American Medical Society for Sports Medicine and the American Orthopedic Society for Sports Medicine: human immunodeficiency virus and other blood borne pathogens in sports. Joint position statement. Am J Sports Med 1995; 23(4):510–4.

57. Zinder SM, Basler R, Foley J, et al. National athletic trainers' association position statement: skin diseases. J Athl Train 2010;45(4):411–28.

58. Sports related skin infections: position statement and guidelines. National Federation of State High School Associations. Available at: http://www.nfhs.org. Accessed December 12, 2010.

59. Fitzpatrick TB, Johnson RA, Wolff K, et al, editors. Cutaneous fungal infections. Color atlas and synopsis of clinical dermatology. 3rd edition. New York: McGraw-Hill; 1997. p. 688–733.

60. Gupta AK, Cooper EA, Ryder JE, et al. Optimal management of fungal infections of the skin, hair, and nails. Am J Clin Dermatol 2004;5:225–37.

61. Brickman K, Einstein E, Sinha S, et al. Fluconazole as a prophylactic measure for tinea gladiatorum in high school wrestlers. Clin J Sport Med 2009;19:412–4.

62. Anderson BJ. The epidemiology and clinical analysis of several outbreaks of herpes gladiatorum. Med Sci Sports Exerc 2003;11:1809–14.

63. Barton SE, Ebel CW, Kirchner JT, et al. The clinical management of recurrent genital herpes: current issues and future prospects. Herpes 2002;9:15–20.

64. Anderson BJ. Managing herpes gladiatorum outbreaks in competitive wrestling: the 2007 Minnesota experience. Curr Sports Med Rep 2008;7(6):323–7.

65. Theos AU, Cummins R, Silverberg NB, et al. Effectiveness of imiquimod cream 5% for treating childhood molluscum contagiosum in a double blind, randomized pilot trial. Cutis 2004;74:134–42.

66. Syed TA, Lundin S, Ahmad M. Topical 0.3% and 0.5% podophyllotoxin cream for self-treatment of molluscum contagiosum in males. A placebo-controlled, double-blind study. Dermatology 1994;189(1):65–8.

67. Habif T. Clinical dermatology. 5th edition. Philadelphia: Elsevier Health Sciences; 2009. Chapter 9.

68. Kazakova SV, Hageman JC, Matava M, et al. A clone of methicillin-resistant *Staphylococcus aureus* among professional football players. N Engl J Med 2005;352(5):468–75.

69. Creech CB, Saye E, McKenna BD, et al. One-year surveillance of methicillin-resistant *Staphylococcus aureus* nasal colonization and skin and soft tissue infections in collegiate athletes. Arch Pediatr Adolesc Med 2010;164(7):615–20.

70. Moellering RC Jr. Current treatment options for community-acquired methicillin-resistant *Staphylococcus aureus* infection. Clin Infect Dis 2008;46:1032–7.

71. Gowitz RJ. The role of ancillary antimicrobial therapy for the treatment of uncomplicated skin infections in the era of community-associated methicillin-resistant *Staphylococcus aureus*. Clin Infect Dis 2007;44:785–7.

72. Harbarth S, Dharan S, Liassine N, et al. Randomized, placebo-controlled, double-blind trial to evaluate the efficacy of mupirocin for eradicating carriage of methicillin-resistant *Staphylococcus aureus*. Antimicrobial Agents Chemother 1999;43(6):1412–6.
73. Garza D, Sungar G, Johnston T, et al. Ineffectiveness of surveillance to control community-acquired methicillin-resistant *Staphylococcus aureus* in a professional football team. Clin J Sport Med 2009;19(6):498–501.
74. Elston DM. How to handle a CA-MRSA outbreak. Dermatol Clin 2009;27:43–8.

Attention-Deficit Hyperactivity Disorder and the Athlete: New Advances and Understanding

Jesse W. Parr, MD*

KEYWORDS

- ADHD • Sports • Thermoregulation • Exercise physiology
- Drug therapy

In recent years there has been an apparent increase in the number of athletes arriving on college campuses with a diagnosis of attention-deficit/hyperactivity disorder (ADHD) and taking medication to treat the ADHD.[1] The active ingredients in these medications include the stimulants amphetamine and methylphenidate (MPH), which seem to have performance-enhancing activity. Furthermore, many athletes have the diagnosis of ADHD made after arriving on college campuses when they begin to struggle academically. Despite an incidence in the general population reported anywhere between 4% and 7%,[2] there seems to be a slightly increased incidence of ADHD in college athletes (Jesse W. Parr, personal observation, June 2, 2010). This brings up several questions[1]: is ADHD a legitimate, medically based condition about which clinicians should be concerned?[2] How is it possible that athletes with ADHD could make it to college and not be diagnosed previously if they really have ADHD?[3] Is the apparent increased incidence of ADHD among college athletes compared with the incidence in the general population legitimate?[4] What, if any, effect is there on sport performance from having a diagnosis of ADHD? And what, if any, effect is there on sport performance and/or thermoregulation from taking medicines used to treat ADHD.[5]

Disclosures: Speaker's Bureau Shire Pharmaceuticals, Speaker's Bureau Lilly Pharmaceuticals. The author is a member of the speaker's bureau for Shire Pharmaceuticals and Lilly Pharmaceuticals.
Department of Pediatrics, Texas A&M Health Science Center, Texas A&M University, College Station, TX, USA
* University Pediatric Association, 1602 Rock Prairie Road, Suite 340, College Station, TX 77845.
E-mail address: jparr@athletics.tamu.edu

Clin Sports Med 30 (2011) 591–610
doi:10.1016/j.csm.2011.03.007
0278-5919/11/$ – see front matter © 2011 Elsevier Inc. All rights reserved.

sportsmed.theclinics.com

THE NATIONAL COLLEGIATE ATHLETIC ASSOCIATION PERSPECTIVE

From the perspective of the National Collegiate Athletic Association (NCAA), the concern with medication for ADHD and sports competition results from the realization that, in recent years, the number of student athletes testing positive for these stimulant medications has increased threefold[1] and, in many cases, there has been inadequate documentation submitted in support of the request for a medical exception to the NCAA banned drug policy. The NCAA bans classes of drugs because they can harm student athletes or they can create an unfair advantage in competition, but some legitimate medications contain substances banned by the NCAA and student athletes may need to use these medicines to support their academics and their general health.

WHAT IS ADHD

The *Diagnostic and Statistical Manual, Fourth Edition* (DSM-IV),[3] of the American Psychiatric Association defines ADHD as a heterogeneous behavioral disorder with multiple possible causes, characterized by problems with inattention or impulsivity/overactivity, or both, causing impairment in all or most areas of life, and not better explained by another mental disorder (eg, autism or mental retardation), with onset in childhood, although symptoms may not be noticed or cause impairment until later in life. The course is persistent rather than episodic, and the characteristics may not always be impairing. Each of these points is discussed in more detail. In the past century, this condition has been called minimal brain damage (1930), hyperactive child syndrome, minimal brain dysfunction, hyperkinetic reaction of childhood, attention-deficit disorder (ADD) with or without hyperactivity, and now ADHD. All of these refer to the same condition.

A Heterogeneous Behavioral Disorder

The clinical characteristics of persons with ADHD vary greatly in character as well as severity, but are manifest as problems with behavior. These problems with behavior may involve difficulty with (1) academics; (2) compliance with scholastic, family, and societal rules; and (3) social relations with peers. The most recognizable symptoms are the overactivity and impulsivity displayed by children with ADHD, but difficulty with inattention is more academically impairing. Evidence is beginning to emerge that some persons with ADHD also have more difficulty with emotional regulation than control subjects.

Multiple Possible Causes

The most frequent cause is heredity, and ADHD is among the most hereditable disorders in humans, with 75% to 80% of its cause being genetic. Several genes involved in the manufacture, packaging, release, and reuptake of the neurotransmitters dopamine (DA) and norepinephrine (NE), as well as genes determining the receptors to these neurotransmitters, seem to be related to the cause of ADHD. The cause of the remainder involves either traumatic brain injury or perinatal events causing injury to the brain areas involved in executive functions.

Characterized by Problems with Inattention and/or Overactivity/Impulsivity

Although not present in all subjects with ADHD, the most recognizable behavioral characteristic is overactivity/impulsivity, most commonly referred to as hyperactivity. Impulsivity is a general tendency to speak and act without reflection on the appropriateness of the activity. These children are frequently referred to their physician early in life for further evaluation after they begin to have behavior problems at home, preschool, or early elementary years. Persons who have only the inattentive variety of ADHD may not come to clinical attention until later in life when the demands of school exceed their compensating strategies. This inattention is confusing because they do not have difficulty paying attention when the task is fascinating. Fascination is different from directed attention toward a task. Fascination involves the reward circuits of the brain, whereas directed attention involves the executive functions of the brain. Executive functions are those processes involved in the brain's self-management[4] and are discussed later. Persons with ADHD may be able to pay attention for hours while playing with fascinating items or video games, as well as during sport, but, when forced to direct attention to more mundane topics, such as academic work, even though their effort is the same as their non-ADHD classmates, their brain simply goes off-task. There is some emerging information to suggest that some persons with ADHD also have more difficulty with emotional regulation than those who do not have ADHD.

Causing Impairment

Each of the characteristics of ADHD occurs to some degree in everyone, but ADHD is diagnosed when these characteristics are severe enough to cause impairment or distress to the affected individual. This impairment may occur at home, at school, on the playground, on the sports field, at work, in relationships, and so forth. Affected persons may also be distressed because they are treated differently by their peers because of their behavior, or the distress may also be experienced by the other members of the household, either parents, siblings, or spouse.[2]

Not Better Explained by Another Mental Disorder

ADHD shares symptoms with other conditions and these must be considered in the differential diagnosis. In general, the most helpful characteristic is the lifetime and persistent nature of the symptoms of ADHD. Although the affected person may not experience impairment caused by ADHD until later childhood, adolescence, or early adulthood, these characteristics have been present all of their lives, which is most problematic in those persons who do not have significant hyperactivity. It is sometimes necessary to look for evidence of inattention in childhood and, although the DSM-IV requires symptoms to be present by 7 years of age, most experts now simply require evidence of symptoms by midadolescence. The inattention and/or hyperactivity are persistent and not remitting. Other conditions that must be considered are autistic spectrum disorders, mood disorders, and learning or language disorders.

Onset in Childhood

As mentioned in previously, the signs and symptoms of ADHD should have onset in childhood, although their impairment may not occur until later in life. Academically, this occurs at the point at which the demands become too great for the child to be successful just by being present in class. This point may occur at any time from later elementary school until college. Children who have problematic overactivity are usually recognized in early elementary school as their behavior begins to disrupt the educational experience of their classmates and as they have difficulty complying with school rules and regimentation.

Symptoms are Persistent, Not Episodic

Persons with ADHD experience unremitting symptoms throughout life. Although bipolar disorder shares numerous symptoms with ADHD, persons with bipolar disorder have remitting symptoms that, although they recur, are not persistent. Other mood disorders may impair attention and schoolwork but they too have a more remitting and recurring nature, whereas ADHD symptoms are persistent through life and in all circumstances.

Characteristics May Not Always be Impairing

In some circumstances, the symptoms and signs of ADHD may offer an advantage. For our ancestors who lived in a more dangerous world, being distractible might have meant noticing danger or opportunities that other more focused members of the community did not. The ability to act without reflection (impulsivity) could offer advantages in responding to danger or in obtaining food. The need to be active would be an advantage in obtaining food for the family. In some sports, impulsiveness corresponds with the quick decision making required of a point guard, quarterback, or baseball catcher.

How is ADHD Diagnosed?

Diagnosis is by a systematic review of the medical, developmental, educational, and behavioral history. This review can be facilitated by using standardized questionnaires or by a structured diagnostic interview. Physical and neurologic examination is also done looking for possible comorbidities that might affect function. Diagnosis is not made by testing. Although ADHD is conceptualized as a disorder of brain executive function, currently there are no neurobiological or neuropsychological tests for ADHD with sufficient sensitivity and specificity to serve as an individual diagnostic test.[5] Although static and functional imaging are useful in detecting group differences between patients with ADHD and controls, imaging studies are not useful in making the diagnosis in an individual patient, and additionally are prohibitively expensive. There has been a recent surge in interest in the use of cognitive electrophysiology, which may provide data that are more sensitive to the diagnosis than cognitive-performance data alone.[6,7] Ultimately, the diagnosis rests on a systematically obtained history using standardized questionnaires.

What is the Underlying Neurobiology?

In the past, ADHD was seen as a socially learned behavioral disorder originating in environmental influences including parenting. It has also been seen as a moral failure in those persons having ADHD. Attempts at treatment emphasized behavioral strategies to change the parenting of the caregiver to cause change in the child. It is now understood that the signs and symptoms of ADHD have a biologic origin caused by problems in the frontostriate circuits of the brain involved in what has come to be known as brain executive functions. Executive functions have been defined by Barkley[4] as "a set of neurocognitive processes that allow for the organization of behavior across time so as to attain future goals... These processes include the ability to inhibit motor, verbal, cognitive and emotional activities. Problems in these areas contribute to deficits in working memory, verbal working memory, planning and problem solving and emotional self-regulation."

The frontostriate circuits connect the dorsolateral prefrontal cortex, the anterior cingulate cortex, the orbitofrontal cortex, cerebellum, and striatum (caudate nucleus and putamen).[8] These circuits receive inputs from association cortices that provide sensory data and a bottom-up influence on attention and behavior, which is influenced by saliency (prominence or conspicuousness), fascination, or interest. The prefrontal cortex provides a top-down influence on attention that could be called directed attention.

Function in these neural networks is influenced by activity at postsynaptic α 2a receptors, DA receptors, and presynaptic reuptake pumps for DA and NE. Activity in these networks is influenced by the levels of DA and NE present. According to a recent model of ADHD, activation of noradrenergic α 2a receptors increases signal transmission within the networks by decreasing postsynaptic signal loss on dendritic spines, whereas DA activation decreases noise in the circuits by decreasing postsynaptic signaling from irrelevant areas. Impaired synaptic transmission adversely influences function in those pathways. There also seem to be influences on the function of these circuits by the expectation of reward. Rapid reward reinforces attention and this may explain why children and adults with ADHD have no difficulty paying attention to video games that produce almost immediate reward for appropriate behavior. Functional magnetic resonance imaging (fMRI) studies by Bush and colleagues[9] showed that, compared with controls, the cognitive division of the anterior cingulate cortex failed to activate during the Counting Stroop test, which is an attention/cognitive interference task known to activate this region of the brain in persons without ADHD (**Fig. 1**).[10]

Ventromedial prefrontal cortex circuits also are involved in emotional regulation and many patients with ADHD have difficulty with proper emotional regulation, which is manifest most commonly with oppositional behavior, irritability, and impulsive explosive temper.

Neuroanatomic Differences

Brain volumetric studies using MRI reveal brain volume differences in areas associated with brain functions that are impaired in ADHD (**Fig. 2**).[4,8,10,11]

Furthermore, MRI studies show abnormalities in white matter tracts involved in these frontostriate circuits.[12–15] Cortical maturation has also been shown to be delayed in subjects with ADHD compared with controls.[8,16–18]

New Conceptualization of ADHD

ADHD is now seen as a problem involving, to a variable degree, the executive control and reward circuits of the brain. It is a behavioral disorder with a biologic explanation based in nonoptimal signal transmission in the brain. As previously noted, it is also coming to be seen to involve problems with regulation of emotion.

ADHD Causes Functional Impairment

There is impairment in the quality of life of persons with ADHD compared with controls. Persons with ADHD have decreased educational attainment, increased risk of divorce, and decreased employment status and household income compared with otherwise similar persons without ADHD.[19] Drivers with ADHD have more motor vehicle accidents and speeding tickets than drivers who do not have ADHD.[20] There is frequent psychiatric comorbidity with ADHD. The lifetime risk of having a substance abuse disorder is increased and the overall rate of substance use disorder in ADHD youth is twice that of control youth.[21] Youth with ADHD are more likely to smoke tobacco, to start smoking at an earlier age, and to have more difficulty with discontinuing tobacco use. There is increased risk of having depression, anxiety disorders, and bipolar disorder compared with controls.[22]

Causes of ADHD

Although some cases of ADHD are acquired through traumatic brain injury or by perinatal insult, ADHD is primarily a hereditable disease. Children born to mothers who smoke tobacco during pregnancy are more likely to have ADHD than children born

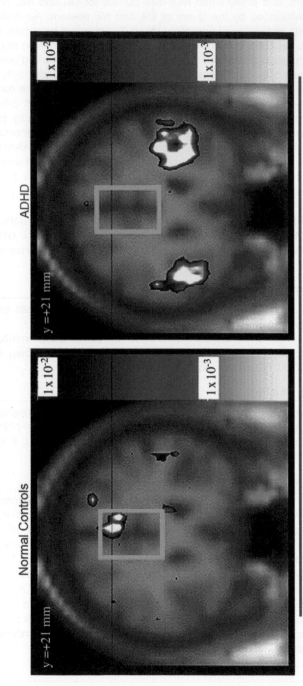

MGH-NMR Center & Harvard-MIT CITP

Fig. 1. Dorsal anterior cingulate cortex (cognitive division) fails to activate in ADHD. Activation of brain during fMRI during the Counting Stroop test, a test affected by ADHD. (*From* Bush G, Frazier JA, Rauch SL. Anterior cingulate cortex dysfunction in attention-deficit/hyperactivity disorder revealed by fMRI and the Counting Stroop. Biol Psychiatry 1999;45(12):1547; with permission.)

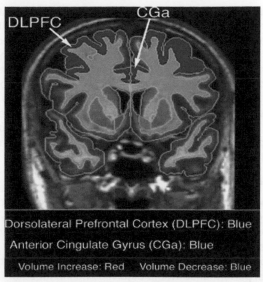

Fig. 2. MRI findings in adult with ADHD. Areas with significant volume decrease in ADHD versus controls on volumetric MRI involving dorsolateral prefrontal cortex (DLPFC) and anterior cingulate gyrus (CGa). (*From* Seidman LJ, Valera EM, Makris N, et al. Dorsolateral prefrontal and anterior cingulate cortex volumetric abnormalities in adults with attention-deficit/hyperactivity disorder identified by magnetic resonance imaging. Biol Psychiatry 2006;60(10):1075; with permission.)

to mothers who do not smoke but are otherwise well matched to the smokers.[23] Numerous studies reveal the hereditability of ADHD to be about 75%.[24] There seem to be multiple genes of small effect that cause great heterogeneity in those with ADHD. These genes primarily are involved in the synthesis, packaging, and release of the catecholamines DA and NE, and with their presynaptic reuptake transporters and postsynaptic receptors.[24] There are other environmental factors that seem to increase the risk of having a child with ADHD, including exposure to organophosphate pesticides and lead.

Incidence in the Population

The incidence in the general population varies but generally is around 5% of the population and is similar on all continents and in all nations.[25] ADHD persists into adulthood and currently most adults who have been diagnosed with ADHD were not diagnosed until adulthood. For reasons that are discussed later, the incidence in athletes may be slightly higher than that in the general population.

How is it that Some Persons with ADHD are not Diagnosed Until College and Young Adulthood?

Persons who have the combined form of ADHD with both overactivity/impulsivity and inattention problems present with symptoms and are usually diagnosed in early elementary school because of the impact of their behavior on the educational environment of other students. Persons who only have clinically significant inattention may not experience obvious impairment until the demands of life and/or school become too complex for compensating strategies. College attendance usually means loss of parental external control and support, which exposes inadequately developed internal control. This loss is sometimes called loss of scaffolding. College students lose their executive secretary, usually called mom, at the same time that the complexity of educational life greatly increases. College is more difficult and requires more sustained effort than high school. Many students diagnosed for the first time with ADHD in college report that high school required little effort to pass. Although the impairment caused by ADHD may not become obvious until college, the characteristics of inattention, disorganization, easy distractibility, and inability to maintain sustained academic effort have been present throughout their scholastic life and can be discovered by systematic questioning. Although DSM-IV requires evidence of symptoms and impairment before age 7 years, most experts require evidence of the symptoms by adolescence.[26]

Athletes with ADHD

A student with good athletic ability and ADHD or any other academic risk factor tends to focus more on areas where they are successful. Most of the positive feedback to the student athlete comes from sports and not from academics. In most students with ADHD, motor function is unimpaired and sports are an outlet for their need to be active. Also, exceptional athletes may be passed along because of their athletic ability even though school performance would otherwise be inadequate.

Fliers and colleagues[27] showed that parents and teachers reported motor coordination problems in about one-third of children with ADHD. These problems persisted into adolescence, but most children with ADHD do not have motor problems. Pitcher[28] showed that, on average, children with ADHD had significantly poorer movement ability than control children, but the results could not be attributed to inattention and concentration problems. Thus, those children with ADHD who do not have motor coordination problems do not have their motor skills impaired by inattention.

Thus, most children with ADHD do not have motor coordination problems, and, particularly if they do not have their ADHD diagnosed, these children have less success in academics, and have more positive interaction with others around sport than academics. As discussed later, ADHD may offer an advantage in some sports activities. Taking all of these circumstances together, children with ADHD who are not motor impaired continue to participate in sports longer than their unaffected peers and develop their sport skills further.

What is the Effect of ADHD on Sport?

Many exceptional athletes have ADHD and, in some circumstances, ADHD may offer advantages. Impulsivity may equate with spontaneity and quick decision making. This connection may be shown by the baseball catcher noting a runner straying too far off base and quickly throwing to pick off the runner, without the delay produced by reflecting on the appropriateness of the activity. Basketball point guards who are good playmakers and football quarterbacks have need of quick decision making, or rather the ability to make a play instantly (impulsively) without reflection. Many athletes report the ability to hyperfocus on enjoyable activities, just as the child may do when playing with enjoyable toys; they are able to block out distractions and focus on the competitive event, as shown by Michael Phelps, the multiple Olympic gold medal winning swimmer, who has ADHD and has legendary ability to do so.

Something which I have noticed but which has not been studied systematically is that athletes with preexisting ADHD who sustain a concussion and undergo repeated computerized neurocognitive testing after the concussion fail to return to baseline scores despite resolution of all symptoms and despite totally normal neurologic examination (Jesse W. Parr, unpublished observation, October 2009). Careful observation during testing bouts by our athletic trainer noted that these athletes had more difficulty sustaining their attention to the testing during the repeated testing bouts compared with athletes without ADHD. On questioning, the ADHD athletes reported that the computerized neurocognitive testing had lost its novelty and they were not interested in the test after 1 postconcussion testing episode. Searches of the medical literature through PubMed failed to find any objective support for this personal observation.

Effect of Sport on ADHD

Kiluk and colleagues[29] showed that children with ADHD who participated in 3 or more sports displayed significantly fewer anxiety or depression symptoms than those who participated in fewer than 3 sports. These differences were not noted in control children who did not have ADHD. Thus, sport participation may improve function in children with ADHD. For children with ADHD, involvement in sports can thus improve their lives far beyond the playing field. Sports can become a haven from the negative feedback they receive in other situations. Children with ADHD may persist in sports participation longer than other children and thus become a larger portion of adolescent and adult athletes than the rate of ADHD occurrence in the general population.

One Institution's Experience

In the 2009 to 2010 academic year, Texas A&M University in College Station (TX) had 701 total NCAA athletes. Fifty of these athletes were taking stimulant medication for ADHD. An uncertain number were taking nonstimulant medication. Those taking stimulants were 7.1% of the total number of athletes. Adding the students taking nonstimulant medication, the total number of athletes at our institution with ADHD was 7% to 9% (author's unpublished observations).

What Medications are Used to Treat ADHD?

Medications used to treat ADHD have an effect on neurotransmission in the frontostriatocerebellar circuits and networks involved in brain executive functions and reward pathways.[30–32] The neurotransmitters that are involved are DA and NE, acting primarily on postsynaptic DA D1 receptors, and noradrenergic α 2a receptors respectively.[32–34] The stimulant drugs MPH and amphetamine block both DA and NE reuptake transporters in the prefrontal cortex and the striatum, and both enhance DA and NE release. This increases the level of neurotransmitter in the synaptic cleft, which improves signaling. Enhancing dopaminergic function seems to decrease the noise level in neural networks, whereas enhancing noradrenergic function seems to increase the strength of the signal by decreasing postsynaptic signal loss. Both of these activities thus improve function in the neural networks involved in executive function and reward. The most bothersome adverse effects of the stimulant drugs for ADHD are decreased appetite, cognitive and/or emotional blunting, and sleep problems. Because of these adverse effects, other nonstimulant medications have been developed. Concern about long-term effect on the brain by stimulant treatment was addressed by a study by Shaw and colleagues,[35] who found that stimulants influence cortical growth in a more normal fashion than would occur in ADHD without stimulant treatment.

The nonstimulant medications used most commonly are atomoxetine (Strattera), guanfacine (Tenex, Intuniv), and clonidine (Catapres, Kapvay), whereas occasionally bupropion (Wellbutrin) and tricyclic antidepressants are used.[36] Atomoxetime selectively blocks the NE transporter in the prefrontal cortex, which increases both NE and DA in the prefrontal cortex, and animal studies show that therapeutic doses of atomoxetine improve prefrontal cortex function through both NE α 2a function and DA D1 actions.

Guanfacine works directly at postsynaptic α 2a receptors in the prefrontal cortex, where it mimics the beneficial effects of NE. When guanfacine occupies the postsynaptic α 2a receptor, it closes the hyperpolarization-activated cyclic nucleotide–gated (HCN) ion channels that dissipate neural signal. This closure enhances signal transmission by decreasing signal loss. Clonidine is less selective for the α 2a receptor than guanfacine and, although it too enhances signaling by decreasing signal loss, its α 2b and 2c functions add significant adverse effects such as sedation and hypotension, and thus it is less useful. All of these nonstimulants have 24-hour durations of action and must be taken daily, and there is usually a delay of several weeks before onset of clinically significant improvement. α 2A Agents frequently are used concurrently with stimulant drugs both to augment their beneficial effect and to diminish the severity of adverse effects on sleep.

The stimulant drugs have a duration of action that varies from 4 to about 12 hours, depending on the preparation (ie, either immediate-release or delayed-release products). **Table 1** shows the differences between the stimulant drugs. In general, the pharmacokinetic profiles are divided into pulse release of active drug (releasing all active drug in a bolus), or smooth release (releasing active drug slowly during a period of time). In general, smooth release causes less subjective awareness of onset of effect (ie, less kicking-in of the drug).

Table 1
Forms of stimulant medication. Pharmacokinetics (PK) means whether released as a bolus (pulse) or released gradually during an extended period of time (smooth)

Stimulant Drugs Available 2011	Duration (h)	Form	Composition	PK
Amphetamine				
Adderall tablet	4	Tablet	Mixture of D,L-amphetamine salts	Pulse
Adderall XR	8–10	Capsule/beads	D,L-Amphetamine mix	Pulse
Vyvanse	12	Capsule/powder	D-Amphetamine prodrug	Smooth
Dexedrine	4–5	Tablet	D-Amphetamine	Pulse
Dexedrine spansule	8	Capsule	D-Amphetamine	Smooth
MPH				
Generic tablet	4	Tablet	D,L-MPH	Pulse
Methylin liquid	4	Liquid	D,L-MPH	Pulse
Ritalin SR	8	Tablet	D,L-MPH	Smooth
Focalin tablet	4–6	Tablet	D-MPH	Pulse
Focalin XR	8–10	Capsule/beads	D-MPH	Pulse
Ritalin tablet	4	Tablet	D,L-MPH	Pulse
Ritalin LA	8	Capsule/beads 50:50	D,L-MPH	Pulse
Concerta	12	Capsule; must swallow intact	D,L-MPH	Smooth
Daytrana	9–12	Transdermal patch	D,L-MPH	Smooth
Metadata CD	8	Capsule beads 30:70		

All capsules except Concerta may be opened and the contents swallowed with food. Concerta should be considered a capsule-shaped tablet.
D- denotes only D optical isomer; D,L- denotes mixture of D and L optical isomers. The D form of the drug is the active component.

The nonstimulant drugs have a delay in onset of benefit from onset of treatment of about 3 to 6 weeks. The reason for this delay is uncertain but probably related to their mechanism of action. They all have 24-hour duration of action, although benefit is greatest in the first 12 hours. They are not schedule II drugs, and thus can be written as regular prescriptions and are refillable. Their primary adverse effects are different from those of the stimulants. Decreased appetite, sleep problems, and cognitive blunting are less likely. Their use is permitted by the NCAA during competition without a therapeutic use exemption (TUE), and is permitted by the World Anti-Doping Association. A recent review by May and Kratochvil[33] summarizes recent advances in pediatric pharmacotherapy for ADHD.

Studies reviewing the effect of supplementation of the diet with ω 3 long-chain polyunsaturated fatty acids (LCPUFAs) such as eicosapentaenoic acid (EPA) and docosahexaenoic acid (DHA) have shown promise in decreasing symptoms of ADHD as well as other childhood developmental disorders.[37–42] Currently, supplemental sources of these ω 3 LCPUFAs are from fish oil as well as single-cell sources of DHA from algae. These ω 3 LCPUFAs are involved in neuronal membrane fluidity and gene expression regulation, and this is postulated to be the mechanism of action. Tobacco smokers with ADHD experience nicotine-related reductions in ADHD symptoms during their everyday lives.[43–45] As stated previously, tobacco smoking during pregnancy increases the risk of ADHD in offspring, so nicotine is somehow involved in ADHD symptoms.

Modafinil (Provigil) is a nonstimulant drug that showed promise in treating ADHD, but revised safety labeling for the drug now includes warnings about the risk of serious Stevens-Johnson syndrome and other serious adverse effects, and thus it is not approved for use in pediatric patients for any indication.

What is the Risk of Substance Abuse in Persons with ADHD Who Take These Drugs?

Patients with ADHD who are not treated have a much greater lifetime risk of recreational drug abuse. Despite persons with ADHD having about twice the lifetime risk of substance use disorder than persons who do not have ADHD, persons with ADHD who are treated with stimulant drugs have the same risk of recreational drug abuse as control subjects. Therefore, stimulant drug treatment, although not protective from substance abuse, does not increase the likelihood of lifetime substance abuse. The reason for the lack of addiction to orally administered stimulant drugs was addressed in a study by Volkow that showed marked differences in the rate of delivery of stimulant drug to the brain and disappearance of the drug from the brain between orally administered and intravenously administered MPH (**Fig. 3**).[46]

When administered intravenously, MPH elicits large and fast DA increases in the brain similar to intravenously administered cocaine, but, when given orally, MPH elicited slow, steady-state increases that did not produce euphoria or a reinforcing effect (desire for another dose). Substance abuse in subjects with ADHD may also be influenced by stimulant treatment of ADHD decreasing the risk of subsequent psychiatric comorbidity and academic failure, both of which predispose to substance abuse.[18]

Unproven or Disproven Therapies

Because of the desire to avoid pharmacologic treatment, several other strategies have been tried in the treatment of ADHD. These therapies lack the degree of scientific support required by the US Food and Drug Administration for approval of currently used ADHD medications. Among these are electroencephalogram biofeedback, elimination diets, megavitamin therapy, sensory integration training, chiropractic skull

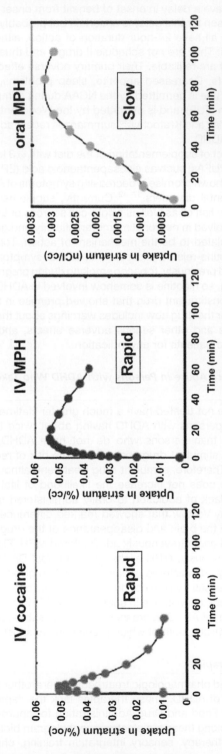

Fig. 3. Rate of drug uptake into the brain. Contrasting rate of uptake and release of oral MPH and intravenous cocaine. Cocaine (IV) and MPH (IV) produce a high but MPH (oral) does not. The slow brain uptake of oral MPH permits effective treatments without a high. (*From* Volkow ND, Ding YS, Fowler JS, et al. Is methylphenidate like cocaine? Studies on their pharmacokinetics and distribution in the human brain. Arch Gen Psych 1995;52(6):461; with permission.)

manipulation, play therapy, and psychotherapy. Social skills training may benefit children whose inattention adversely affects their social interaction.

What is the Effect of ADHD Medication on Sports Activity?

In 1980, Chandler and Blair[47] showed significant increases in knee extension strength, acceleration, anaerobic capacity, time to exhaustion during exercise, pre-exercise and maximum heart rates, and time to exhaustion during maximal oxygen consumption (Vo_2 max) testing after administration of 15 mg of dextroamphetamine versus placebo. Most of the information to answer this question has been obtained in the past decade through studies of fatigue rather than an attempt to systematically investigate the effect of ADHD drugs on exercise.

In 2006, Meeusen and colleagues[48] in Belgium published a review in which they reported that, when fatigue was initially conceptualized to be a central nervous system phenomenon rather than a peripheral phenomenon, serotonin was believed to be involved. The original fatigue hypothesis suggested that exercise induced an increase in extracellular serotonin in several brain regions, which contributed to fatigue. This hypothesis was consistent with the well-known effects of serotonin on lethargy and loss of motivation. They showed there was no evidence from studies to support this hypothesis but that emerging evidence from work investigating physiologic responses to amphetamine does show a role for DA in development of fatigue. They stated that "fatigue during prolonged exercise clearly is influenced by a complex interaction between peripheral and central factors."

In 2002, Watson and colleagues[49] studied the effect of the dual DA/NE reuptake inhibitor bupropion on exercise performance in temperate and warm environments. They showed enhanced performance in warm conditions but not in temperate conditions. The subjects produced greater power output and had higher core temperatures without perception of increased effort or thermal stress.

Swart and colleagues[50] in 2009 studied 8 cyclists who were given either MPH or placebo acutely and studied the effect on their performance. These subjects did not have ADHD and were not regular users of stimulant drugs. They showed that, after acute administration of MPH, cyclists cycled 32% longer than with placebo before power output fell to 70% of starting value. At the time the placebo trials terminated, athletes on MPH had higher power outputs, oxygen consumptions, heart rates, ventilatory volumes, and blood lactate concentrations, although electromyogram activity remained the same. Their conclusions were that "acute administration of MPH, which affects both DA and NE, allowed subjects to have increased power output and to resist fatigue suggesting that endurance performance is not only limited by peripheral fatigue but by the central nervous system."

Roelands and colleagues,[51] also in Belgium, published in 2008 a study of 8 well-trained cyclists. The subjects were given either placebo or 20 mg of MPH 1 hour before exercise. They were exercised either in a temperate (18 degrees centigrade) environment or a warm (30 degrees centigrade) environment. Before the study, the maximum work (Wmax) was determined for each cyclist. During the study, the cyclists cycled for 60 minutes at 55% Wmax followed by a time trial (TT). MPH did not influence TT performance at 18 degrees but TT was 16% faster in 30-degree environment in those subjects taking the MPH than those taking placebo. Core temperature was higher at rest and throughout the TT in those taking MPH and cycling in the warm environment, reaching values in excess of 40 degrees, a temperature previously associated with onset of fatigue, because presumably the brain attempts to protect itself from excessive heat. Throughout the study in the warm environment, heart rate was higher in those subjects who were given MPH than in those given placebo. However, for subjects given MPH, perceived exertion and perceived thermal stress were not changed from their perception during the placebo trial. Their conclusion was that "methylphenidate may potentially increase the risk of developing heat illness during exercise in individuals taking drugs of this nature."

These studies were done in individuals who consumed the stimulant drug acutely, but were not regular users. What is known about the effect of regular use of ADHD medications on exercise? Roelands and colleagues[52] studied the effect of chronic administration of bupropion on exercise in the heat and in a temperate environment. Bupropion also blocks reuptake of both DA and NE. Cyclists were studied in both the temperate and warm environment after taking bupropion or placebo for 10 days. Chronic administration of bupropion did not influence TT performance but significantly increased core temperature, although less than during acute ingestion. Their conclusion was that "it seems that chronic administration of bupropion results in adaptation of central neurotransmitter homeostasis, resulting in different response to the drug than when given acutely."

In 2008, Roelands and colleagues[53] studied the effect of reboxetine, a pure NE reuptake inhibitor, similar to atomoxetine, in 9 healthy, well-trained cyclists. They too exercised in both temperate and warm environments. They showed decreased power output and exercise performance at both 18 and 30 degrees centigrade. Their conclusion was that DA reuptake inhibition was the cause of the increased exercise performance seen with drugs that affect both DA and NE (MPH, amphetamine, and bupropion).

Mahon and colleagues[54] studied exercise performance in boys who had ADHD and who regularly took stimulant medicine. They studied 14 boys who were exercised at 25 W, 50 W, 75 W and a peak exercise test on days when they took their stimulant medication and on days when they took placebo. Submaximal heart rate was higher by 8 to 13 beats per minute during the medication trials. Oxygen uptake, respiratory exchange ratio, and perceived exertion were similar in trials with stimulant and with placebo. However, in those trials following administration of placebo, oxygen uptake, heart rate, and work rate were attenuated compared with trials with stimulant, but their perceived exertion was not changed. There was decreased exercise performance in 6 of the 13 boys. Their conclusion was that "without stimulant medication, physiologic responses at peak exercise are attenuated in some but not all boys with ADHD who regularly take stimulant medication."

Perhaps of some value are studies of 3,4-methylenedioxymethamphetamine (MDMA; known as ecstasy) and heat production. Mills and colleagues[55] in 2004 showed that "norepinephrine release mediated by MDMA creates a double edged sword of heat generation through activation of uncoupling protein (UCP3) along with adrenergic stimulation and loss of heat dissipation through sympathetic nervous system mediated vasoconstriction." Mitochondrial uncoupling proteins separate oxidative phosphorylation from ATP synthesis with energy dissipated as heat. It is unknown whether NE release by ADHD medications causes this as well.

Crystal meth is methamphetamine. The methyl group added to amphetamine is responsible for the potentiation of effects compared with the related compound amphetamine, rendering the substance more lipid soluble and easing transport across the blood-brain barrier, and also prolonging its effect. MDMA shares the same characteristics as methamphetamine. Parrot in 2004,[56] seeking to understand the observed effects of MDMA used at dances called "raves" in which users consume MDMA and dance to rhythmical music on hot, crowded dance floors, showed in rats that hot, noisy, overcrowded conditions potentiated the stimulatory effects of the drug. In humans, the similar conditions of the dance floor may potentiate the effect as well. Of concern is whether hot, noisy, crowded conditions of competition also potentiate the effects of stimulants other than MDMA, such as MPH and amphetamine.

Summary of Effects of ADHD Medication on Exercise Performance

Emerging data from fatigue studies suggests that acute administration of stimulants benefits aerobic exercise and seems to be mediated through effects on DA function in the brain. This benefit is associated with potential risk of thermal stress injury, thus athletic trainers and coaches need to know which athlete is taking ADHD medications and watch them more carefully than others for heat illness. Chronic administration of ADHD medications may decrease the acute effect. Little is known on the effect of ADHD medications on anaerobic function.

In numerous conversations with athletes with ADHD who take stimulant medication I find that there is no consistent answer to whether they believe that their medicine benefits or impairs athletic performance. Some athletes find that their medicine helps them maintain their focus in practice but adversely effects performance in competition. Baseball pitchers commonly use their medicine when charting pitches but most do not benefit from medicine when on the mound. Some athletes state that they perform better in competition while on stimulant medicine because of the relief of their ADHD symptoms, whereas others complain that spontaneity is impaired when on stimulant medicine. Thus, I leave it to each individual athlete to determine when to use their medicine. The impairment of ADHD is not just in academic areas, and no one asks athletes with impaired vision to play their sport without corrective lenses because it is not an academic pursuit.

Cardiac Safety and ADHD Medications

There is no greater risk of sudden cardiac death in patients taking stimulants for ADHD than in comparable populations without ADHD not taking stimulants. The risk that exists is that of sudden cardiac death related to having structural heart disease. The American Heart Association (AHA) made a recommendation that all persons who were to receive stimulant drugs for ADHD should have an electrocardiogram (EKG) beforehand.[57] This statement was countered by the American Academy of Child and Adolescent Psychiatry and the American Academy of Pediatrics and was subsequently retracted by the AHA.[57–59] The current recommendation is that doing an EKG before treatment is fraught with the same problems related to doing EKG as part of sports preparticipation examination. The cost of following up abnormal EKGs and the lack of adequate providers to appropriately read pediatric EKGs in athletes limit the usefulness and cost-effectiveness. The consensus currently is to do a careful history and physical examination and to do an EKG and cardiology referral only in those persons with significant abnormalities on the history and physical.[60] I currently use the questions on the sports preparticipation examination related to cardiac risk as part of my assessment of persons being evaluated for ADHD.[59]

TUE

The NCAA allows a TUE for stimulant use by athletes with adequate documentation of diagnosis of ADHD and evidence of continued follow-up, and the drug may be present at the time of competition. This policy is because of the dual role of student and athlete in NCAA competition. According to the NCAA:

> *The documentation should include a comprehensive clinical evaluation, recording observations and results from ADHD rating scales, a physical examination and any lab work, previous treatment for ADHD, and the diagnosis and recommended treatment. The physician can provide documentation of the above either with a cover letter and attachments or provide the medical record. This documentation should be kept on file in the athletics department until such time that the student*

athlete tests positive for the stimulant. A simple statement from the prescribing physician that he or she is treating the student athlete for ADHD with said medication IS NOT adequate documentation.

The expectation is that for many student-athletes, the evaluation and initiation of treatment likely began during grade school. Documentation of that evaluation, along with the history of treatment and current prescription, should be submitted by the student-athlete to their sports medicine staff upon matriculation.

An annual follow-up with the prescribing physician is the minimum standard, and that can be reflected in a letter from the physician or a copy of the medical record, with written indication of the current treatment.[1]

However, in events sanctioned by national governing bodies, which are not part of the NCAA competition, World Anti-Doping Association and United States Anti-Doping Association (USADA) rules apply.[61] Stimulant drugs are banned during competition unless the athlete has obtained a TUE beforehand. The process requires similar documentation as does the NCAA process, with the added criterion that an athlete initially diagnosed as a young adult must obtain a second opinion from an ADHD specialist.[62] The application is reviewed by the USADA Therapeutic Use Exemption Committee and ruled on individually. Further detailed information is available on the USADA Web site. This USADA TUE policy went into effect on January 1, 2010.[63] Professional sports also allow a therapeutic use exemption, but the number of professional athletes diagnosed with ADHD and treated with stimulants is not public knowledge.

SUMMARY

ADHD is currently understood to be a disorder involving problems in the executive function circuits and reward circuits in the brain. These functional abnormalities cause inhibitory deficits, behavioral and cognitive problems, as well as reward delay aversion, which produce significant impairment in the lives of individuals affected by ADHD. These impairments may be relieved by medication in most circumstances, but these medications may have impacts on sports performance as well as on thermoregulation and, thus, affected individuals who use ADHD medications should be monitored closely by athletic staff, particularly when exercising in hot environments.

For varying reasons, athletes may not be diagnosed with ADHD until after arriving at college. Furthermore, there may be legitimate reasons why there might be an increased incidence of ADHD in college and professional athletes. ADHD and ADHD medications have a variable effect on sports performance and no generalization about ADHD and sport participation can be made. There are no absolutes. Let athletes discover and decide on the best sport for themselves, and also allow athletes to decide whether to take their medication for sports activities based on their personal experience.

REFERENCES

1. NCAA Banned Drugs and Medical Exceptions Policy Guidelines Regarding Medical Reporting for Student-Athletes with Attention Deficit Hyperactivity Disorder (ADHD) Taking Prescribed Stimulants. The National Collegiate Athletic Association. 2009. Available at: www.ncaa.org. Accessed November 9, 2010; and Addendum to the January 2009 Guidelines Q&A March 2009. Accessed November 9, 2010.
2. Kessler RC, Adler L, Barkley R, et al. The prevalence and correlates of adult ADHD in the United States: results from the National Comorbidity Survey Replication. Am J Psychiatry 2006;163(4):716–23.
3. Diagnostic and statistical manual of mental disorders. Text revision. 4th edition. Arlington (VA): American Psychiatric Publishing, Inc; 2000.

4. Barkley RA. Differential diagnosis of adults with ADHD: the role of executive function and self-regulation. J Clin Psychiatry 2010;71(7):e17.
5. Boonstra AM, Osterlaan J, Sergeant JA, et al. Executive functioning in adult ADHD: a meta-analytic review. Psychol Med 2005;35(8):1097–108.
6. Liotti M, Pliszka SR, Perer R, et al. Electrophysiological correlates of response inhibition in children and adolescents with ADHD: influence of gender, age and previous treatment history. Psychophysiology 2007;44(6):936–48.
7. Kuntsi J, McLoughlin G, Asherson P. Attention deficit hyperactivity disorder. Neuromolecular Med 2006;8(4):461–84.
8. Emond V, Joyal C, Poissant H. Structural and functional neuroanatomy of attention-deficit hyperactivity disorder (ADHD) [abstract]. Encephale 2009; 35(2):107–14 [in French]. Accessed November 9, 2010.
9. Bush G, Frazier JA, Rauch SL, et al. Anterior cingulated cortex dysfunction in attention-deficit/hyperactivity disorder revealed by fMRI and the Counting Stroop. Biol Psychiatry 1999;45(12):1542–52.
10. Castellanos RX, Lee PP, Sharp W, et al. Developmental trajectories of brain volume abnormalities in children and adolescents with attention-deficit/ hyperactivity disorder. JAMA 2002;288:1740–8.
11. Seidman LJ, Valera EM, Makris N, et al. Dorsolateral prefrontal and anterior cingulated cortex volumetric abnormalities in adults with attention-deficit/ hyperactivity disorder identified by magnetic resonance imaging. Biol Psychiatry 2006;60(10):1071–80.
12. Silk TJ, Vance A, Rinehart N, et al. White-matter abnormalities in attention deficit hyperactivity disorder: a diffusion tensor imaging study. Hum Brain Mapp 2009; 30(9):2757–65.
13. Makris N, Buka SL, Biederman J, et al. Attention and executive systems abnormalities in adults with childhood ADHD: a DT-MRI study of connections. Cereb Cortex 2008;18(5):1210–20.
14. Bush G, Valera EM, Seidman LJ. Functional neuroimaging of attention-deficit/ hyperactivity disorder: a review and suggested future directions. Biol Psychiatry 2005;57(11):1273–84.
15. Konrad K, Eickoff SB. Is the ADHD brain wired differently? A review on structural and functional connectivity in attention deficit hyperactivity disorder. Hum Brain Mapp 2010;31(6):904–16.
16. Shaw P, Eckstrand K, Sharp W, et al. Attention-deficit/hyperactivity disorder is characterized by a delay in cortical maturation. Proc Natl Acad Sci U S A 2007;104(49):19649–54.
17. Shaw P, Rabin C. New insights into attention-deficit/hyperactivity disorder using structural neuroimaging. Curr Psychiatry Rep 2009;11(5):393–8.
18. Biederman J, Monuteaux MC, Spencer T, et al. Do stimulants protect against psychiatric disorders in youth with ADHD? A 10-year follow-up study. Pediatrics 2009;124(1):71–8.
19. Biederman J, Faraone SV, Spencer TJ, et al. Functional impairments in adults with self-reports of diagnosed ADHD: a controlled study of 1001 adults in the community. J Clin Psychiatry 2006;67:524–40.
20. Barkley RA, Murphy KR, Dupaul GI, et al. Driving in young adults with attention deficit hyperactivity disorder: knowledge, performance, adverse outcomes, and the role of executive functioning. J Int Neuropsychol Soc 2002;8(5):655–72.
21. Biederman J, Wilens TE, Mick E, et al. Does attention-deficit hyperactivity disorder impact the developmental course of drug and alcohol abuse and dependence? Biol Psychiatry 1998;44(4):269–73.

22. Biederman J, Monuteaux MC, Mick E, et al. Young adult outcome of attention deficit hyperactivity disorder: a controlled 10-year follow-up study. Psychol Med 2006;36(2):167–79.

23. Milberger S, Biederman J, Faraone SV, et al. Is maternal smoking during pregnancy a risk factor for attention deficit hyperactivity disorder in children? Am J Psychiatry 1996;153(9):1138–42.

24. Faraone SV, Perlis RH, Doyle AE, et al. Molecular genetics of attention-deficit/hyperactivity disorder. Biol Psychiatry 2005;57(11):1313–23.

25. Faraone SV, Sergeant J, Gillberg C, et al. The worldwide prevalence of ADHD: is it an American condition? World Psychiatry 2003;2(2):104–13.

26. Faraone SV, Biederman J, Spencer T, et al. Diagnosing adult attention deficit hyperactivity disorder: are late onset and subthreshold diagnoses valid? Am J Psychiatry 2006;163(10):1720–9.

27. Fliers E, Rommelse N, Vermeulen SH, et al. Motor coordination problems in children and adolescents with ADHD rated by parents and teachers: effects of age and gender. J Neural Transm 2008;115(2):211–20.

28. Pitcher TM. Fine and gross motor ability in males with ADHD. Dev Med Child Neurol 2003;45(8):525–35.

29. Kiluk BD, Weden S, Culotta VP. Sport participation and anxiety in children with ADHD. J Atten Disord 2009;12(6):499–506.

30. Bush G, Spencer TJ, Holmes J, et al. Functional magnetic resonance imaging of methylphenidate and placebo in attention-deficit/hyperactivity disorder during the multi-source interference task. Arch Gen Psychiatry 2008;65(1):102–14.

31. Rubia K, Halari R, Cubillo A, et al. Methylphenidate normalizes activation and functional connectivity deficits in attention and motivation networks in medication-naïve children with ADHD during a rewarded continuous performance task. Neuropharmacology 2009;57(7–8):640–52.

32. Arntsen AF. Toward a new understanding of attention-deficit hyperactivity disorder pathophysiology: an important role for prefrontal cortex dysfunction. CNS Drugs 2009;23(Suppl 1):33–41.

33. May DE, Kratochvil CJ. Attention-deficit hyperactivity disorder: recent advances in paediatric pharmacotherapy. Drugs 2010;70(1):15–40.

34. Brennan AR, Arntsen AF. Neuronal mechanisms underlying attention deficit hyperactivity disorder: the influence of arousal on prefrontal cortical function. Ann N Y Acad Sci 2008;1129:236–45.

35. Shaw P, Sharp WS, Morrison M, et al. Psychostimulant treatment and the developing cortex in attention deficit hyperactivity disorder. Am J Psychiatry 2009; 166(1):58–63.

36. Wigal SB. Efficacy and safety limitations of attention-deficit hyperactivity disorder pharmacotherapy in children and adults. CNS Drugs 2009;23(Suppl 1):21–31.

37. Johnson M, Ostlund S, Fransson G, et al. Omega-3/omega-6 fatty acids for attention deficit hyperactivity disorder: a randomized placebo-controlled trial in children and adolescents. J Atten Disord 2009;12(5):394–401.

38. Richardson AJ, Montgomery P. The Oxford-Durham study: a randomized, controlled trial of dietary supplementation with fatty acids in children with developmental coordination disorder. Pediatrics 2005;115(5):1360–6.

39. Richardson AJ. Omega-3 fatty acids in ADHD and related neurodevelopmental disorders. Int Rev Psychiatry 2006;18(2):155–72.

40. Germano M, Meleleo D, Montorfano G, et al. Plasma, red blood cells phospholipids and clinical evaluation after long chain omega-3 supplementation in

children with attention deficit hyperactivity disorder (ADHD). Nutr Neurosci 2007; 10(1–2):1–9.

41. Schuchardt JP, Huss M, Stauss-Grabo M, et al. Significance of long-chain poly-unsaturated fatty acids (PUFAs) for the development and behavior of children. Eur J Pediatr 2010;169(2):149–64.
42. Kirby A, Woodward A, Jackson S, et al. Childrens' learning and behavior and the association with cheek cell polyunsaturated fatty acid levels. Res Dev Disabil 2010;31(3):731–42.
43. Gehricke JG, Whalen CK, Jamner LD, et al. The reinforcing effects of nicotine and stimulant medication in the everyday lives of adult smokers with ADHD: a prelim-inary examination. Nicotine Tob Res 2006;8(1):37–47.
44. Gehricke JG, Hong N, Whalen CK, et al. Effects of transdermal nicotine on symp-toms, moods, and cardiovascular activity in the everyday lives of smokers and nonsmokers with attention-deficit/hyperactivity disorder. Psychol Addict Behav 2009;23(4):644–55.
45. Gehricke JG, Louglin SE, Whalen Ck, et al. Smoking to self-medicate attentional and emotional dysfunctions. Nicotine Tob Res 2007;9(Suppl 4):S523–36.
46. Volkow ND, Ding YS, Fowler JS, et al. Is methylphenidate like cocaine? Studies on their pharmacokinetics and distribution in the human brain. Arch Gen Psych 1995;52(6):456–63.
47. Chandler JV, Blair SN. The effect of amphetamines on selected physiological components related to athletic success. Med Sci Sports Exerc 1980;12(1):65–9.
48. Meeusen R, Watson P, Hasegawa H, et al. Central fatigue: the serotonin hypoth-esis and beyond. Sports Med 2006;36(10):881–909.
49. Watson P, Hasegawa H, Roelands B, et al. Acute dopamine/norepinephrine reup-take inhibition enhances human exercise performance in warm, but not temperate conditions. J Physiol 2005;565(pt 3):873–83.
50. Swart J, Lamberts RP, Lambert MI, et al. Exercising with reserve: evidence that the central nervous system regulates prolonged exercise performance. Br J Sports Med 2009;43:782–8.
51. Roelands B, Hasegawa H, Watson P, et al. The effects of acute dopamine reup-take inhibition on performance. Med Sci Sports Exerc 2008;40(5):879–85.
52. Roelands B, Hasegawa H, Watson P, et al. Performance and thermoregulatory effects of chronic bupropion administration in the heat. Eur J Appl Physiol 2009;105(3):493–8.
53. Roelands B, Goekint M, Heyman E, et al. Acute norepinephrine reuptake inhibi-tion decreases performance in normal and high ambient temperature. J Appl Physiol 2008;105(1):206–12.
54. Mahon AD, Stephens BR, Cole AS. Exercise responses in boys with attention deficit/hyperactivity disorder: effects of stimulant medication. J Atten Disord 2008;12(2):170–6.
55. Mills EM, Rusyniak DE, Sprague JE. The role of the sympathetic nervous system and uncoupling proteins in the thermogenesis induced by 3,4-methylenedioxy-methamphetamine. J Mol Med 2004;82(12):787–99.
56. Parrott AC. MDMA (3,4-methylenedioxymethamphetamine) or ecstasy: the neuro-psychobiological implications of taking it at dances and raves. Neuropsychobiol-ogy 2004;50(4):329–35.
57. Vetter VL, Elia J, Erickson C, et al. Cardiovascular monitoring of children and adolescents with heart disease receiving stimulant drugs: a scientific statement from the American Heart Association Council on Cardiovascular Disease in the

Young Congenital Cardiac Defects Committee and the Council on Cardiovascular Nursing. Circulation 2008;117(18):2407–23.

58. Pliszka S, American Academy of Child and Adolescent Psychiatry, Work Group on Quality Issues. Practice parameter for the assessment and treatment of children and adolescents with attention-deficit/hyperactivity disorder. J Am Acad Child Adolesc Psychiatry 2007;46(7):894–921.

59. American Academy of Pediatrics, Committee on Quality Improvement, Subcommittee on Attention-Deficit/Hyperactivity Disorder. Clinical practice guideline: diagnosis and evaluation of the child with attention-deficit/hyperactivity disorder. Pediatrics 2000;105(5):1158–70.

60. Denchev P, Kaltman JR, Schoenbaum M, et al. Modeled economic evaluation of alternative strategies to reduce sudden cardiac death among children treated for attention deficit/hyperactivity disorder. Circulation 2010;121(11):1329–37.

61. TUEs and Medical Declarations; TUEs FAQs. United States Anti-Doping Agency. Available at: http://www.usada.org/tue-faq. Accessed November 9, 2010.

62. USADA Policy for Therapeutic Use Exemptions and Declaration of Use. United States Anti-Doping Agency. Available at: http://www.usada.org/tue-policy/. Accessed September 17, 2010.

63. Documentation to support a Therapeutic Use Exemption application for stimulants to treat ADD/ADHD. United States Anti-Doping Agency. Available at: http://www.usada.org/files/pdfs/TUEhowto.pdf. Accessed September 17, 2010.

Psychiatric and Neuropsychological Issues in Sports Medicine

Ali Esfandiari, PhD, Donna K. Broshek, PhD*,
Jason R. Freeman, PhD

KEYWORDS

• Athletes • Psychiatry • Psychology • Neuropsychological
• Therapy

Athletes are a unique sample of the population when it comes to mental health issues. Being an athlete carries strong stereotypes that have been demonstrated to influence behavior based on the principle of stereotype–threat.[1] One common stereotype is that athletes are somehow immune to the mental health concerns that may affect the general population. Athletes frequently feel they must live up to the stereotyped image of being tough minded and less sensitive to life's challenges. However, athletes face a number of challenges that predispose them to be particularly at risk for mental health issues.[2]

This article reviews the current knowledge about athletic training room psychiatric/ psychological issues and how to recognize them, and provides an initial framework for how to manage them. There is some focus on psychiatric issues involved in collegiate sports medicine environments, because the majority of research on athletes has been conducted in the college population. Much of this information generalizes to other athletic settings as well. Greater awareness of these problems, empirical research, and education about mental health issues in the sports medicine community are clearly needed.

ATHLETES AND STRESS

Although participation in athletics has itself been demonstrated as a buffer to stress,[3,4] intercollegiate athletes often face stressors that traditional college students do not experience.[5] Most prominently, student–athletes face the daunting task of balancing

---

The authors have nothing to disclose.
Neurocognitive Assessment Laboratory, Department of Psychiatry & Neurobehavioral Sciences, University of Virginia School of Medicine, PO Box 800203, West Complex, 1300 Jefferson Park Avenue, Charlottesville, VA 22908-0203, USA
* Corresponding author.
E-mail address: broshek@virginia.edu

Clin Sports Med 30 (2011) 611–627
doi:10.1016/j.csm.2011.03.002
0278-5919/11/$ – see front matter © 2011 Elsevier Inc. All rights reserved.

class time, practice time, competition time, study time, social activities, and an exhausting travel schedule. These extreme time demands can relegate self-care activities to the backseat. In addition to adjusting to the dual demands of athletics and academics, athletes can struggle to manage the heightened visibility among their peers that may provide unwanted attention. Additionally, they can face unique pressures from family members who may be overinvolved in their athletic endeavors, and they may have to deal with injuries, playing time issues, and conflicts with coaches and teammates.[5] The transition from high school to college itself can be especially stressful for athletes.[6] Since most college athletes were star players on their high school teams and in their home community, a reduced role on the team can be a challenge. When it comes time to end their college careers, athletes often have to cope with finishing their career in the sports spotlight in addition to graduation,[7] or face the evolving stressor of coping with professional sports, an environment with exacting demands and a narrow margin for error.

Today's athletes, even during the formative athletic experiences of junior high school, are exposed to longer seasons and longer training hours. Such trends may contribute to a narrowing of social supports and structures at later points in life. They also require considerable energy to manage multiple relationships with coaches, families, teammates, peers, classmates, friends, and the larger community.[8] As athletic performances begin to occupy an increasingly significant proportion of their self-identity, athletes must learn ways of successfully coping with the pressure of maintaining high levels of performance. Athletes may worry that coaches, the community, and the media will criticize or abandon them if their performance decreases.

At the collegiate level, there appears to be a great contrast between nonathlete students and their athletic counterparts. Extracurricular activities expand social opportunities for the former, but the time commitment of collegiate athletics limits availability for special activities and other campus resources that could widen learning, support, and social interaction opportunities.[9] This can have a profound impact on the psychological functioning of athletes at all levels, and these community stressors should be considered in evaluating the presence, severity, and nature of emotional distress as it presents in the training room. The context of such issues is critically important in directing athletes to the appropriate treatment. A medication evaluation for an athlete who has psychosocial stress or isolation may prove insufficient. Strong consideration should also be given to referring for supportive or directive therapy to examine and manage the behavioral and environmental contributors to the distress.

The college setting has offered a unique situation for examining athletic stressors. There is a widening athletic divide, particularly for the recruited collegiate athlete, from the general student population, especially at many elite academic institutions.[9] Recruited athletes as a group tend to have lower Scholastic Aptitude Test (SAT) or American College Testing (ACT) scores than their walk-on athlete and nonathlete counterparts, and their academic and socioeconomic backgrounds may not prepare them in areas typically emphasized in college. Recruited athletes tend to earn a substantially lower grade point average in college, and this difference is especially pronounced among recruits in high-profile sports (namely football and men's basketball), as they have been shown to average between the 19th and 23rd percentiles in grade point average (GPA).[9] Lower-profile male recruits (29th to 37th percentiles) and female recruits (39th to 46th percentiles) also showed a difference relative to same-gender nonathletes, although to a lesser degree. These difference hold up even when controlling for time demands, majors, and preadmission test scores.

Since maintaining academic eligibility is a central responsibility of being a student–athlete, grades can frequently become a primary trigger for emotional distress. This can especially be the case for athletes who were recruited primarily for their athletic talent despite deficiencies in their academic preparation. Distress can grow exponentially if academic underperformance threatens athletic eligibility and jeopardizes a scholarship. Such situations can lead athletes to feel they are being exploited for their athletic talents, which can lead the athlete to perceive a lack of loyalty by the university or college after they have completed their eligibility.[8] These athletes may experience resentment that the school benefited economically from their athletic exploits, and subsequently may feel used and abandoned if they are no longer able to compete. According to Parham,[8] this experience is more frequent for African American athletes, resulting in anger, bitterness, and hurt. The same feelings may occur in professional athletes who are traded and feel discarded by the city where they contributed to the sports franchise and charitable activities in the community. These perceived stressors, unsupported, might lead to clinically significant depression, anxiety, aggression, conflict in the community, or to substance abuse.

ATHLETES AND MENTAL HEALTH

Given the myriad of stressors faced by athletes, the environment for triggering mental health issues is ripe. However, mental health issues may not always be noticed or addressed appropriately by athletic staff. One reason is that athletes may minimize any apparent signs of perceived weakness. Also, symptoms can sometimes fly under the radar due to the acceptance, at times even promotion of many behaviors (eg, black–white thinking, hyperactivity, perfectionist drives) within athletic culture. Sometimes symptoms of psychiatric illness that would be identified and diagnosed in the general population are attributed to overtraining or physical exhaustion in the athletic setting.[10]

The first point of contact for athletes with mental health issues is typically the sports medicine professionals and team physicians who must consider psychological concerns when coordinating care for injured athletes. Athletes may initially present with concomitant physical conditions, with exaggerated physical ailments that mask underlying mental health issues, or without any specific physical complaints. Danish and colleagues[11] established criteria to recognize athletes at risk. Identifiable warning signs may include an excessive preoccupation with a quick return following an injury, denial of the negative effects of an injury, excessive guilt concerning the failure to contribute to the team, and isolating or withdrawing from social support (eg, teammates) and other commitments.

Athletes without physical complaints may sometimes present after much encouragement from teammates, athletic trainers, or coaches. Sometimes coaches will force the player to address mental health issues if it becomes too disruptive to the team. Despite efforts by the National Alliance for the Mentally Ill (www.nami.org), considerable stigma still exists regarding psychiatric and psychological conditions, a stigma that remains an even stronger barrier for athletes to seek help given the athlete stereotypes mentioned previously. Reframing therapy to appeal to an athlete's competitive behavior—by naming it "performance enhancement"—can help improve an athlete's willingness to seek services.[12]

PREVALENCE AND INCIDENCE

Despite the clear evidence that athletes face unique challenges that impact mental health, the research literature on psychiatric issues in athletes remains surprisingly limited. A recent article by Reardon and Factor[13] systematically reviewed the existing literature on psychiatric disorders in athletes. Although early evidence revealed that athletes seek psychotherapy less often than their nonathlete counterparts,[14,15] the consensus is that athletes experience psychiatric disorders at the same rate as the general population,[16] although some disorders, namely eating disorders, substance abuse, and attention-deficit hyperactivity disorder (ADHD)—are seen more frequently in athlete populations. The relationship between an athlete and his or her psychiatric disorder can take many forms.[17] An athlete may obtain a high level of success despite the disorder, as in the case of an athlete who slugs through his or her depressive symptoms and still manages to perform well. Athletes can also be drawn toward specific sports as an outlet for their disorder or as a means of coping with their disorder; an example would be the ADHD athlete who is drawn to lacrosse for its constant barrage of stimulation. Finally, an athlete may have a psychiatric illness worsened by the sport itself. Someone with underlying depression may have their symptoms exacerbated by a poor performance, a critical coaching staff, an exhausting schedule, and the perception of letting down their teammates. The following sections review some of the most prevalent psychiatric conditions faced by the general community and athletes.

DEPRESSION

Sadness and frustration are normal reactions to a lost match, a bad practice, or a nagging injury. Many people may use the word depression to explain these kinds of transient feelings, but clinical depression is distinct from ordinary feelings of sadness or frustration. Clinical depression is marked by pervasive and chronic feelings of intense sadness and hopelessness along with other emotional and physiologic symptoms that generally last for a period of at least 2 weeks but often much longer. Common symptoms of depression can include dysphoria, tearfulness, social withdrawal, anhedonia, changes in cognitive ability, and disruptions in sleep, appetite, energy, motivation, or libido. Suicidal ideation is a concerning symptom in more severe cases. **Box 1** lists characteristics distinguishing normal transient feelings of being down from clinical depression.

At any given time, approximately 5% of the US population suffers from depression, with lifetime prevalence rates ranging from 10% to 25% for women, and 5% to 12% for men.[18] While some studies have reported that high school athletes tend to have fewer depressive symptoms than nonathletes,[19,20] studies performed with collegiate athletes tend to suggest that student–athletes have rates of depression that are in line with the general population.[16,21,22] Others, however, have demonstrated that rates of depression may be lower in athletes.[23] Within the athlete population, females, freshmen, and injured athletes tend to be more likely to exhibit symptoms of depression.[22]

A bout of depression in athletes can be triggered by a failure in competition, overtraining, an injury, by circumstances unrelated to athletics, or there may be no salient trigger. Depression can sometimes arise during the high-risk period of transition during the end of one's collegiate career. This tends to be a time of heightened emotional distress as athletes evaluate their athletic career accomplishments against their initial expectations. It may be difficult to cope with the feelings of unrealized potential, just as it is difficult to let go of the identity of being an athlete. This period can be especially distressing for athletes who have a strong psychological attachment to their sport, a history of devotion to their sport to the exclusion of other activities, and a higher level of success in the sport.[8]

Diagnosing depression in athletes is difficult, because athletes may deny low mood. Additionally, other physical symptoms may be attributed to overtraining. Depression may be perceived as an admission of weakness in the athletic community. To avoid

> **Box 1**
> **Distinguishing between feeling down and clinical depression**
>
> - Normal blues
>   - Short-lived (less than 2 weeks, typically much less)
>   - Not pervasive (may feel content much of the time)
>   - Capable of keeping up with responsibilities and life demands
>   - Low energy does not persist
>   - Still derive pleasure from activities
> - Depressive disorder
>   - Lasts more than 2 weeks
>   - Pervasive sadness for much of day
>   - Significantly interferes with functioning
>   - May adversely affect sleep, appetite, energy, and cognitive ability
>   - Anhedonia
>   - In severe cases, self-harm or suicidal ideation

the stigma of appearing depressed, athletes may present with symptoms of insomnia, fatigue, and other somatic complaints, or there may be a marked shift in their academic performance and a growing dislike of their sport. The symptoms of depression overlap significantly with overtraining syndrome (OTS). Often athletes who would otherwise receive a diagnosis of depression in medical settings are more likely to receive a diagnosis of overtraining in athletic settings.[10] Since many symptoms of overtraining are similar to those of clinical depression, if athletes present with issues related to burnout in their sports, further evaluation is recommended to determine whether the issue is actually depression.

Treatment for depression can involve psychotherapy, pharmacologic agents, or both. In the authors' experience, the behavioral component of depression treatment is often handled by the structure provided by athletics. Since the athlete often must continue to be present for practice, remain physically active, and continue to interact with teammates, behavioral activation is generally not needed while the athlete remains active in his or her sport. On the other hand, athletes in general can benefit greatly from brief cognitive interventions that target rigid cognitions that may be contributing to low mood.

BIPOLAR DISORDER

Bipolar disorder involves the presence of depressive episodes and at least 1 manic (type 1) or hypomanic (type 2) episode.[18] Manic episodes can include elevated, irritable, or expansive mood lasting more than 1 week, with accompanying inflated self-esteem, diminished need for sleep, increased or pressured speech, racing thoughts, excessive distractibility, increased goal-directed activity, or excessive indulgence in hedonic activities with a high risk of adverse consequences (eg, spending, gambling, sexual indiscretion, substance abuse). The lifetime prevalence rate is between .5% and 1.6%, and age of onset is typically in the late teens to early 20s, with men typically having an earlier onset than women.[18] A family history of mood disorder significantly increases the risk of developing bipolar disorder. Although there are no known prevalence data regarding bipolar disorder in athletes, it is an important diagnostic consideration for high school, college, and early professional athletes presenting with evidence of the aforementioned symptoms.

EATING DISORDERS

Eating disorders are marked by abnormal eating habits that may involve either insufficient or excessive food intake to the detriment of an athlete's physical and emotional health. They are believed to occur at a higher rate in athletic populations, especially in females.[16] In the athletic training room, consideration of how coaches' and parents' behaviors and expectations influence negative eating patterns may be essential to ensuring a good plan of care.

OVERTRAINING

The defining symptom of OTS is a sudden drop in performance and training capacity that is precipitated by training stress with insufficient recovery. Capacity to train is typically impacted for a period of at least several weeks to several months. Illness, injury, and psychosocial stressors are not the primary cause of this decrease in performance capacity. Additional symptoms can be both physical and psychological and may include a washed-out feeling or lack of energy, soreness or general aches and pains, changes in mood (most frequently irritability or depressive symptoms), changes in appetite and sleep, decreased immunity, and a compulsive desire to exercise.

The prevalence of OTS has not been adequately studied. Survey research suggests that 7% to 21% of endurance athletes annually suffer with OTS, and that up to 64% of elite distance runners report experiencing OTS at least once in their careers.[24] In a study sample of 231 teen swimmers, 34.6% reported at least 1 occurrence of OTS persisting for an average of 3.6 weeks.[25] Athletes who have a history of OTS appear to be at greater risk of developing OTS again, with 1 study demonstrating a 91% chance of return within 3 years.[24]

As previously mentioned, there are many similarities between OTS and major depression. Disruptions in mood are related to training load; as training load intensifies so do mood disruptions.[26] The similarities between OTS and depression—and their possible co-occurrence—can create difficulties in making an accurate diagnosis.[27] As such, referral to a mental health clinician should be a component of treatment for OTS. Since the primary component of treatment for OTS is an extended period of time off from the sport (often several weeks), prevention is a preferred goal. However, there have been no reliable markers for early detection of OTS. Nederhof and colleagues[28] conducted a set of meta-analyses and determined that impaired psychomotor speed may be a potential indicator that could serve as a future marker for preventing OTS. Additionally, some research has found that OTS may be prevented by altering the training loads of athletes in response to mood changes.[24]

ANXIETY DISORDERS

Anxiety is commonplace in athletes as they face internal and external demands to perform at an optimal level and often under intense pressure. While a certain level of anxiety is needed for successful athletic performances (see Hanin's[29] review of what constitutes these levels), optimal levels of anxiety are sometimes exceeded and can begin to interfere with athletic performance. **Box 2** lists characteristics that distinguish between normal anxiety (or nerves) and clinically significant anxiety.

> **Box 2**
> **Distinguishing between nerves and clinically significant anxiety**
>
> - Normal anxiety
>   - Temporary
>   - Situational (eg, before a performance)
>   - Does not interfere with performance or functioning in daily life
>   - Worries are manageable
> - Anxiety disorder
>   - Chronic (lasts more than 6 months)
>   - Pervasive
>   - Significantly interferes with functioning
>   - Worries are difficult to manage
>   - Stimuli associated with anxiety are avoided or endured with distress

No known studies examine the prevalence rates of anxiety disorders in athletes. However, there is no reason to believe that prevalence rates vary significantly from the general population. Prevalence rates of anxiety disorders in the general population vary from as low as 1.5% for panic disorder up to a high of 12% to 13% for specific phobia, social phobia, and generalized anxiety disorder.[18]

Although much attention has been devoted to performance-related anxiety in athletes, by comparison the studies on anxiety disorders are minimal and have been primarily focused on social anxiety. As its name implies, social anxiety is anxiety about social situations, interactions with others, and being evaluated by other people. Norton and colleagues[30] studied 180 students and found that social anxiety can generalize to competitive athletics, particularly for those athletes in individual sports. The results suggest that socially anxious athletes may experience increased evaluation anxiety if they have difficulty living up to their own expectations or those of their family. Storch and colleagues[31] studied 398 college students (105 intercollegiate athletes) and found that female athletes were more likely to express symptoms of social anxiety compared with female nonathletes and both male athletes and nonathletes.

Anxiety in the athlete can take various forms, but telltale signs that anxiety is becoming a clinical issue include athlete dread of going to practice, avoidance of sports-related activities altogether, or enduring these activities only under duress. Often an athlete will first present for treatment with concerns about performance anxiety, and upon further investigation it is revealed that their initial symptoms represent a more pervasive disorder. Indeed, a full third of performance anxiety cases can be attributed to manifestations of generalized anxiety disorder, and 10% to 15% of patients who have performance anxiety have comorbid major depressive disorder.[32] The development of a therapeutic alliance with team psychologists can facilitate the discovery of the source of an athlete's anxiety. Escape and avoidance behaviors—and ritualistic behavior meant to allay anxiety—can often serve to maintain or exacerbate anxiety. Behavioral approaches remain the treatment of choice for athletes who experience anxiety symptoms. Exposure-based treatments, along with relaxation training, are often sufficient to lessen levels of anxiety to target levels. Athletes with problematic anxiety often experience more significant anxiety from their own perceived failure to live up to expectations rather than judgments about their performance that they receive from others. Challenging these thoughts—through therapeutic intervention known as cognitive therapy—can help change the patterns of thinking that contribute to anxiety, replacing them with more positive and realistic thoughts.

ADHD

ADHD consists of two main symptom clusters: inattention and hyperactivity/disinhibition. Either or both can be primary. Inattention involves difficulty in sustaining attention to the task at hand, while hyperactivity/disinhibition involves a deficiency in the ability to suppress excessive motor activity, impulsive behaviors, or otherwise delay gratification. ADHD has been primarily studied in children, and is believed to affect between 2% to 5% of American school-aged children, with boys outnumbering girls by between 4 to 9 times.[18]

Prevalence of ADHD in athletes is less well understood. In one survey given to 870 intercollegiate athletes, Hiel and colleagues[33] found the rate of diagnosed ADHD to be 7.3%, which is higher than the prevalence rates for the general population. Distribution of ADHD athletes tends to be disproportionate; the highest levels are seen in football players (17.5%), and the lowest in track and field (4.4%). These data support the anecdotal experiences in the authors' clinic, in that ADHD tends to be more prevalent in the athletic community than in the general population. As some have hypothesized, one rationale is that those with ADHD are drawn to physical activity,[16] especially sports that are fast-paced and stimulating.[34] Some have further hypothesized that athletes with ADHD tend to be especially attracted to sports that have a higher degree of unpredictability, sports which Michael Stebeno[35] labels as providing continuous chaos, where athletes need to consistently react to multiple sources of stimulation. Conversely, athletes with ADHD are less apt to thrive in slow-paced sports that require extended concentration and focus over long periods. These preferences may help explain the disproportionate distribution of ADHD athletes across sports.

An athlete with untreated ADHD may often be singled out by a coach who is unfamiliar with the disorder. Athletes with ADHD can often act before thinking and can demonstrate impulsive behavior on and off the field. They may be easily distracted, especially during lulls in the game or during idle time in practice. They may experience low frustration tolerance and difficulty with repetitive tasks. Coaches who mistakenly attribute these behaviors as signs of disrespect may often single out the athlete with ADHD for negative consequences. As such, a successful intervention may include educating the coach on ADHD, its effects, and how to best keep the athlete engaged on the field.

Freshman collegiate athletes with untreated ADHD may struggle to juggle the combination of heightened academic and athletic pressures at the college level. This may be one reason why athletes with ADHD are at particular risk to engage in problematic drinking behavior.[36] When an athlete demonstrates ADHD symptoms, referral for a comprehensive neuropsychological or psychoeducational evaluation should be conducted as early as possible in the athlete's college career. Once formally diagnosed, the appropriate accommodations can be made through the university disability office. Often these academic accommodations will include extra time for taking examinations, special testing environments with reduced distractions, assistance with note taking, and distribution of class content in different formats. Additional information regarding ADHD is provided in a dedicated article in this issue.

PSYCHOTROPIC MEDICATION

Prescribing psychotropic medications for athletes is more complicated than prescribing for the general population, because it requires an understanding of the demands of an athlete's sport, how the medication might affect the athlete's health during grueling physical exertion (eg, increased heart rate, dehydration), and whether the medication will be allowed under the governing guidelines of his or her sport. Anecdotal experience suggests that physicians working with athletes have reservations about using medications to treat psychiatric symptoms because of the lack of empirical evidence in the athlete population; this hesitancy may lead to psychiatric symptoms being undertreated. Additionally, many athletes may be hesitant to take medication for several reasons, most prominently that it may undermine their performance, threaten their sense of self-sufficiency, or for fear that medication might affect their sport eligibility.

A 1999 survey of the members of the International Society for Sports Psychiatry (ISSP) revealed that the majority of prescribers attempted to minimize certain side effects that would be considered problematic in the athletic population.[37] Specifically, 84% of respondents attempted to avoid sedating effects; 62% attempted to minimize extrapyramidal effects, and 58% tried to minimize tremors. While this survey provided important information, it should be interpreted with caution given the low response rate (25%) and small number of overall respondents (N = 19).

For depression, the prescription of choice (63%) tends to be fluoxetine, with venlafaxine (21%), bupropion (11%), and other selective serotonin reuptake inhibitors (SSRIs) (16%) being less often considered. Fewer than 5% reported using clomipramine, fluvoxamine, nefazodone, and paroxetine. The preference for fluoxetine is because of its activating properties and lower risk of weight gain. One study of college athletes demonstrated that fluoxetine had no effect on anaerobic capacity, muscle strength, power, or fatigue, suggesting that fluoxetine is not likely to have an impact on athletic performance.[38] However, in one study by Meeusen and colleagues,[39] endorphins increased significantly less with exercise when an SSRI was administered. In both studies, however, there were serious limitations in experimental design, which limits external validity.

For mood stabilizers, valporic acid (VPA) was the preferred medication, used by 58% of respondents in the ISPP survey.[37] VPA is preferred over lithium, because it is less sedating, less likely to cause weight gain, less likely to cause tremor, and levels of the drug are not altered by dehydration. The most commonly prescribed anxiolytic was buspirone, used by 37% of respondents. Benzodiazepines were generally avoided because of concerns about sedation, dependence, impaired reflexes and balance, and cognitive impairment. Of those that chose to prescribe benzodiazepines, 32% used alprazolam and 26% used lorazepam because of their short half-life and rapid therapeutic effect.

Stimulants are the most common treatment for ADHD, and of athletes formally diagnosed with ADHD, 94% take some form of medication.[33] Of those athletes taking medication, 25% are under the effects of medication while participating in their sport.[33] The prescribing physician needs to be especially careful when prescribing stimulants to athletes. Many athletes now fall under strict new policies that require extensive documentation that demonstrates the student–athlete has undergone a comprehensive clinical assessment to diagnose ADHD and is being monitored routinely for use of the stimulant medication. A detailed discussion of stimulant use is included in a dedicated article in this issue.

SUBSTANCE ABUSE

Despite stringent drug testing requirements within college and professional sports, substance abuse continues to be a pervasive problem. When compared with nonathletes, intercollegiate athletes are more likely to report higher rates of alcohol and drug use or abuse and are more likely to engage in binge drinking and suffer negative consequences (eg, criminal charges, academic trouble, risky behaviors) related to alcohol.[40] Consistent with the general population, alcohol is the most frequently abused substance in athletics,[16,41] although athletes may also use marijuana, cocaine or other illegal substances, as well as prescribed medications such as psychostimulants, anxiolytics, and pain medications despite random drug testing. Alcohol abuse may be harder to detect, since it is not a banned substance.

In college, drinking is viewed as a normative experience, and particular team cultures may promote a culture of drinking.[42] The most salient sign that substance use has become a problem is when there is a pattern of use in the face of repeated negative consequences, whether they are team suspensions, academic or personal failings, or criminal offenses. Additional signs of an addictive disorder include tolerance and withdrawal symptoms, using more of a substance than intended, and difficulty with cutting back on use.

A National Collegiate Athletic Association (NCAA) study of athletes in 30 different sports at 991 schools that yielded 13,914 responses[41] revealed that alcohol was the most widely used substance in the preceding year (85%) followed by cannabis (28.4%), and smokeless tobacco (22.5%). Prevalence of use was higher in Division II and III programs, likely owing to more stringent policing in Division I schools. Men were significantly more likely than women to use the following substances: anabolic steroids, smokeless tobacco, ephedrine, marijuana, psychedelics, and cocaine. The only drugs that did not show a gender differential were alcohol and amphetamines. Caucasian athletes were more likely to report use of amphetamines, ephedrine, alcohol, smokeless tobacco, and psychedelics than African American athletes or individuals from other racial or ethnic backgrounds. There were no significant differences among racial or ethnic groups in their use of anabolic steroids, cocaine/crack, or marijuana/hashish.

Athletes face enormous pressure to compete, even when injured. For professional athletes, the pressure to compete with pain may have significant economic consequences as well. As a result, athletes may be at particular risk for abusing analgesics and drugs that enhance performance. In one study of 563 student athletes,[43] 62% of responders indicated that they used painkilling drugs to alleviate pain or soreness after tougher workouts, 55% after routine workouts, and 29% indicated they saw no problems with using these medications during competitions to reduce their pain. Males were more likely to view painkilling drugs as acceptable. Athletes were more likely to obtain painkilling drugs from friends (60%), teammates (58%), and parents (50%) than from their athletic trainer (38%) or physician (14%), further raising the risk of abuse potential. These results reveal the need for education about the appropriate use of medications and about nonmedication alternatives. Sports medicine teams should have a clear policy about the use of such medications, and communicate directly and frequently with coaches and athletes about this policy (eg, not prescribing narcotic pain relievers just to tolerate pain and remain in competition).

Anabolic steroids are used by 1.2% of Division I athletes,[41] and lifetime use in athletes is estimated to be around 3.3%. These rates are considered to be higher than nonathletes.[44,45] One college-based study found that 12% of current intercollegiate nonsteroid-using student-athletes who participated in strength sports would use anabolic steroids to improve their athletic performance if they would guarantee success and if the athletes could be assured of not testing positive for use.[46] In comparing athletes who use anabolic steroids to those who do not, 23% of users experienced major psychiatric issues, including 12% with psychotic symptoms.[47]

CONCUSSION

A concussion is defined as a trauma-induced alteration in mental status that may or may not involve loss of consciousness. It is the most frequent type of head injury that occurs in sports.[48] Recovery from concussion varies by individual and by the severity of the concussion. Depending on the severity of the concussion, the athlete may experience numerous psychological symptoms such as irritability, depression, and anxiety.[49,50] Management of concussions should therefore be evaluated and managed on a case-by-case basis. Ideally, a concussion program would administer preseason baseline neuropsychological testing so that athletes who sustain a concussion can have their postinjury testing compared with their own baseline performance.[49-52] If symptoms of concussion last for more than 5 to 10 days, consultation with a neurologist and neuropsychologist may be beneficial for managing symptoms, enhancing recovery, and making return-to-play decisions.

PSYCHOLOGICAL REACTION TO INJURY

Participation in competitive sports places high demands on an athlete's body, making the risk of injury ever present.[53] The Centers for Disease Control and Prevention (CDC) estimate that high school athletes experience injuries at a rate of 2.4 injuries per 1000 athletic exposures, with injury rates being highest for football (4.36 per 1000) and other contact sports.[54] Depending on the severity of an injury, athletes may experience psychological reactions ranging from frustration and anger to clinical levels of anxiety, depression, and even grief. As many as 24% of athletes report significant emotional difficulties such as depression or anxiety following an injury, particularly in the first 4 to 8 weeks after the injury.[55] In fact, the stages of psychological reaction to injury may mimic the pattern of grief in response to loss[56] and can include the stages of denial, anger, bargaining, depression, and acceptance.[57]

To examine the course of psychological changes in response to injury, Leddy and colleagues[58] conducted a prospective study of emotional functioning in 343 Division IA male college athletes in 10 different sports. Measures of depression, anxiety, and self-concept were administered during preseason physicals. Athletes who were injured were given these measures again within one week of their injury, along with a randomly selected noninjured athlete. The measures were readministered to both the injured and noninjured athletes at a follow-up 2 months after the injury assessment. The results revealed that still-injured athletes and those who had recovered from an injury had greater depression and anxiety and lower self-esteem compared with noninjured athletes. Although many of the injured athletes experienced mild depression, 12% of those athletes who had sustained an injury had scores on the Beck Depression Inventory in the clinically significant range that merited psychological intervention. Training room medical staff should be aware of the potential psychological consequences of injuries and refer those athletes who have significant emotional distress to appropriate mental health personnel.

Research suggests that psychological factors can play a role in injury even before the injury occurs. Some research has demonstrated that psychological variables, including personality, emotional state, life stressors, and coping skills, can influence an athlete's susceptibility to injury.[59] In a recent review of 40 empirical studies, 85% of studies demonstrated some type of positive relationship between life stress and injury risk.[60] In one study, anxiety and ineffective coping skills were found to be predictive of injury risk in a sample of adolescent soccer players.[61] Although research in this area is still in its infancy, further research on the role psychological factors play in injury etiology may prove useful in eventually developing preventative interventions aimed at lowering an athlete's injury risk profile.

Social support plays a critical role in an athlete's coping with injury. An athlete's recovery from injury can be enhanced if he or she maintains a connection to the competitive environment and stays involved with the team in some fashion.[56,62] As previously noted, teammates often compose the majority of an athlete's support network. Therefore, an injury can engender fear of losing status with the team and losing primary sources of social support. Injured athletes who lose contact with their team and coaches may begin thinking that they were previously valued only for their athletic ability and not as individuals. Negative thoughts may occur, such as "I am valued only for my athletic ability, and since I can no longer perform, I am worthless." Left untreated, athletes with this cognitive style are at risk for depression. Intervention should focus on challenging these all-or-nothing cognitions and fostering a self-image that includes positive characteristics of identity outside of athletics. Treating the depressive reaction will enable the athlete to have increased motivation to participate more readily in the rehabilitation process.

ROLE OF THE MENTAL HEALTH PROFESSIONAL

Given the dearth of research on the prevalence of psychiatric distress and treatment in the sports medicine community, there is still much to learn. Foremost, available data do not include diagnoses based upon agreed-upon criteria (eg, *Diagnostic and Statistical Manual of Mental Disorders*[18]), and it is not clear how such diagnoses are made in sports medicine clinics. Second, although knowing how frequently mental health conditions present in clinics is important, there is still no clear study of the true prevalence rate of specific mental health conditions in athletes. Third, it is not evident how often sports medicine clinics employ consultation with mental health professionals, including psychiatrists, psychologists, and licensed counselors. Although stigma might make such referrals difficult, effective incorporation of such professionals as part of the sports medicine team may normalize symptoms, decrease anxiety, and increase education regarding the identification and treatment of mental health issues.

Because accurate diagnosis is essential for treatment, it is critical that athletic trainers receive adequate training in the recognition of serious psychiatric and psychological disorders. Glick and Horsfall[12] eloquently state that the key to a good evaluation is differentiating the cause of difficulties from their effects. There is often a strong interaction between the stress and dysfunction in the athletic world and the social/interpersonal world. Knowing an athlete well and developing rapport becomes critical to teasing apart how these issues relate to one another, and to determining as much as possible if 1 area of functioning (or dysfunction) is the trigger for more pervasive difficulties. In this sense, this is often a true chicken-and-egg question. Athletes often develop a close and trusting relationship with their athletic trainer, and may disclose information about personal difficulties. Occasionally, such disclosures may reveal more serious problems, and the athletic trainer should listen carefully to the athlete and offer several options for the athlete's consideration.[63] Ideally, the athletic trainer should encourage the athlete to talk to the team physician or an appropriate mental health professional.

Referral to an appropriate mental health specialist may be necessary to most appropriately assess a psychiatric or psychological condition and to develop an integrated treatment plan. At the University of Virginia, clinical neuropsychologists serve as consultants, providing mental health services, educational or neuropsychological evaluations, and concussion management for student athletes. This system allows for an integrated and seamless provision of services with clearly defined lines of communication between the neuropsychologists and sports medicine clinic staff. Because many of the mental health issues facing athletes are complex adjustment issues, psychological services are typically highly effective, particularly cognitive behavioral therapy and active problem-solving approaches.

Team physicians often feel comfortable prescribing psychotropic medications after consulting with a clinical psychologist/neuropsychologist for cases that are straightforward and without concerning comorbidity. For athletes who have more complex psychiatric histories and multiple comorbid psychiatric disorders, a referral can be made to a psychiatrist. Typically, if medications are prescribed, the athletes maintain some level of follow-up with the clinical psychologist, in addition to the team physician, to monitor response and any adverse effects. Psychotherapy in and of itself is wide-ranging in terms of follow-up. For uncomplicated issues, athletes may be seen for as little as one session. In other cases, they may be seen for several years. Predictably, this depends upon the presenting issues, complexity of the problem, the stability of the support network, and the number and nature of their psychosocial stressors. Consistent with the authors' experience, Begel[64] reports that athletes often desire immediate results, and single-session psychotherapeutic interventions are not uncommon.

One of the most important issues to clarify when referring to mental health professionals is confidentiality. Given their involvement with multiple personnel on the field and in the athletic training room (eg, head coach, assistant coaches, athletic trainers, physicians, compliance officers, and administrators) and their often high-profile status, it is critically important that the athletes have a confidential relationship with their therapist. Although it may be necessary for the mental health professional to report on adherence to therapy to ensure appropriate follow-up, the content of any therapy sessions must be confidential from other members of the athletic community. Privacy issues must be addressed directly, both within the sports medicine clinic and between the therapist and athlete. Any limits to confidentiality must be discussed with the athlete at the first meeting. For example, in the authors' sports medicine program, all athletes who have eating disorders are treated using a team approach that involves the therapist, nutritionist, team physician, and medical director. Although sensitive information disclosed to the therapist is kept confidential, athletes are informed that medical issues such as laboratory results and nutritional status will be discussed among the team. If the therapist is aware of behavioral issues that might be affecting medical adherence, these issues may be discussed among the group as well. Psychological issues such as developmental history, family dynamics, or body image concerns discussed with the therapist are kept confidential. As with all therapy patients, imminent safety threats to self (ie, suicidal intent) or others are not kept confidential, and prompt action is taken to ensure the safety of those concerned. In such cases, the minimal amount of disclosure needed to assure safety is provided.

In addition to clinical neuropsychologists, clinical psychologists, and psychiatrists, other mental health professionals, such as licensed clinical social workers and licensed counselors, may also provide appropriate interventions. It is critically important to ensure that the mental health professionals have experience with psychopathology, differential diagnosis of psychiatric disorders, an understanding of normal developmental issues, and experience with the unique pressures faced by amateur and professional athletes. Although access to mental health professionals may not always be immediately available to the athletic training room, other resources may be of assistance. For instance, mental health screening can be incorporated into health management programs within the training room. Information about screening programs for depression and anxiety, such as the QPR (Question, Persuade, Refer) and Jed Foundation Ulifeline, can be found on the mental health issues link of the NCAA Web site at www.ncaa.org/health-safety.

SUMMARY

Mental health issues may be a significant aspect of athlete presentation in the sports medicine clinic, complicating the management of medical issues and independently creating prominent patient care concerns. Depression/mood disorders, anxiety disorders, substance abuse, adjustments to injury, eating disorders, and other psychological disturbances may be subtle or obvious, but require good general clinical skills and awareness to assess the complex interplay among personality, medical, and environmental factors. Although it is thought that the frequency of such psychiatric issues in athletes generally parallels the incidence and prevalence of psychiatric issues in the general population, there has been little empirical study of just how prominent these issues are, or how to most effectively treat them in athletes of varying age and ability. Stigma and lack of education may obfuscate discussion and identification of mental health problems, and may impede referrals to appropriate psychological or psychiatric specialists for treatment. In addition, discussion of confidentiality, any limits of confidentiality, and the safeguard of this trust is essential to optimizing collaborative and integrated care.

Further investigation of how sports medicine clinics assess and manage these issues will permit a more systematic evaluation of various treatment approaches to better care for and protect the mental health, and overall health, of athletes. To facilitate this goal, collaboration of sports medicine professionals with psychiatrists, psychologists, and other mental health professionals can improve communication, debunk the myths associated with mental health care, and promote specialized care within this important area of functioning. In designing this collaboration, sports medicine physicians or athletic trainers often have the closest rapport with athletes, and the vote of confidence given to mental health consultants is critical to establish hope and trust in athletes regarding the potential benefits of such treatment. The power of psychological well-being cannot be overemphasized. Fostering psychological health along with physical health by integrating mental health resources into the routine management of athletes is increasingly vital to their pursuit of excellence.

REFERENCES

1. Dee TS. Stereotype threat and the student–athlete. National Bureau of Economic Research Working Paper Series; 2009. Available at:http://www.nber.org/papers/w14705. Accessed March 12, 2011.
2. Watt SK, Moore JL III. Who are student athletes? New Dir Student Serv 2001;93:7–18.
3. Scully D, Kremer J, Meade MM, et al. Physical exercise and psychological well being: a critical review. Br J Sports Med 1998;32:111–20.
4. Hudd S. Stress at college: effects on health habits, health status, and self-esteem. Coll Student J 2000;34(2):217–27.
5. Kimball A, Freysinger VJ. Leisure, stress, and coping: the sport participation of collegiate student–athletes. Leisure Sci 2003;25:115–41.
6. Pritchard ME, Wilson GS, Yamnitz B. What predicts adjustment among college students? J Am Coll Health 2007;56(1):15–21.
7. Richard S, Aries E. The division III student–athlete: academic performance, campus involvement, and growth. J Coll Student Dev 1999;40(3):211–8.
8. Parham WD. The intercollegiate athlete: a 1990s profile. Couns Psychol 1993; 21(3):411–29.

9. Bowen WG, Levin SA. Reclaiming the game: college sports and educational values. Princeton (NJ): Princeton University Press; 2003.
10. Schwenk TL. The stigmatization and denial of mental illness in athletes. Br J Sports Med 2000;34(1):4–5.
11. Danish SJ, Petitpas AJ, Hale BD. Psychological interventions: a life development model. In: Murphy SM, editor. Sport psychology interventions. Champaign (IL): Human Kinetics; 1995. p. 19–38.
12. Glick ID, Horsfall JL. Diagnosis and psychiatric treatment of athletes. Clin Sports Med 2005;24(4):771–81.
13. Reardon CL, Factor RM. Sport psychiatry: a systematic review of diagnosis and medical treatment of mental illness in athletes. Clin Sports Med 2010;40(11):961–80.
14. Pierce RA. Athletes in psychotherapy: how many, how come? J Am Coll Health Assoc 1969;17(3):244–9.
15. Carmen LR, Zerman JL, Blaine GB Jr. Use of the Harvard Psychiatric Service by athletes and nonathletes. Ment Hyg 1969;52:134–7.
16. Burton RW. Mental illness in athletes. In: Begel D, Burton RW, editors. Sport psychiatry: theory and practice. New York: WW Norton; 2000. p. 61–81.
17. Baum AL. Sport psychiatry: how to keep athletes in the game of life, on or off the field. Curr Psychiatry 2003;2(1):51–6.
18. American Psychiatric Association. Diagnostic and statistical manual of mental disorders, fourth edition, text revision. Washington, DC: American Psychiatric Association; 2000.
19. Oler MJ, Mainous AG III, Martin CA, et al. Depression, suicidal ideation, and substance use among adolescents. Are athletes at less risk? Arch Fam Med 1994;3(9):781–5.
20. Brand S, Gerber M, Beck J, et al. High exercise levels are related to favorable sleep patterns and psychological functioning in adolescents: a comparison of athletes and controls. J Adolesc Health 2010;46(2):133–41.
21. Donohue B, Covassin T, Lancer K, et al. Examination of psychiatric symptoms in student athletes. J Gen Psychol 2004;131:29–36.
22. Yang J, Peek-Asa C, Corlette JD, et al. Prevalence of and risk factors associated with symptoms of depression in competitive collegiate student athletes. Clin J Sport Med 2007;6:481–7.
23. Armstrong S, Oomen-Early J. Social connectedness, self-esteem, and depression symptomatology among collegiate athletes versus nonathletes. J Am Coll Health 2009;57(5):521–6.
24. Raglin JS, Kentta G. A psychological approach toward understanding and preventing the overtraining syndrome. In: Echemendia RJ, Moorman III CT, editors. Praeger handbook of sports medicine and athlete health; Volume 3 Psychological perspectives. Santa Barbara (CA): Praeger; 2011. p. 63–76.
25. Raglin JS, Sawamura S, Alexiou S, et al. Training practices and staleness in 13–18-year-old swimmers: a cross-cultural study. Pediatric Sports Med 2000;12:61–70.
26. Morgan WP, Costill DL, Flynn MG, et al. Mood disturbance following increased training in swimmers. Med Sci Sports Exerc 1988;20(4):408–14.
27. Armstrong LE, VanHeest JL. The unknown mechanism of the overtraining syndrome: clues from depression and psychoneuroimmunology. Sports Med 2002;32:185–209.
28. Nederhof E, Lemmink K, Visscher C, et al. Psychomotor speed: possibly a new marker for overtraining syndrome. Sports Med 2006;36:817–28.
29. Hanin YL. Individual zones of optimal functioning (IZOF) model: emotions-performance relationship in sport. In: Hanin YL, editor. Emotions in sport. Champaign (IL): Human Kinetics; 2000. p. 65–89.

30. Norton PJ, Burns JA, Hope DA, et al. Generalization of social anxiety to sporting and athletic situations: gender, sports involvement, and parental pressure. Depress Anxiety 2000;12:193–202.
31. Storch EA, Storch JB, Killiany EM, et al. Self-reported psychopathology in athletes: a comparison of intercollegiate student–athletes and nonathletes. J Sport Behav 2005;28:86–98.
32. Powell DH. Treating individuals with debilitating performance anxiety: an introduction. J Clin Psychol 2004;60:801–8.
33. Heil J, Hartman D, Robinson G, et al. Attention-deficit hyperactivity disorder in athletes. Available at: http://coaching.usolympicteam.com/coaching/kpub.nsf/v/adhd. Accessed November 10, 2002.
34. Barkley RA. Attention-deficit hyperactivity disorder: a handbook for diagnosis and treatment. 2nd edition. New York: Guilford; 1998.
35. Stabeno M. The ADHD affected athlete. Victoria (Canada): Trafford; 2004.
36. Wilens T, Biederman J, Mick E, et al. Attention deficit hyperactivity disorder (ADHD) is associated with early onset substance use disorders. J Nerv Ment Dis 1997;185:475–82.
37. Baum AL. Psychopharmacology in athletes. In: Begel D, Burton RW, editors. Sports psychiatry: theory and practice. New York: WW Norton; 2000. p. 249–59.
38. Parise G, Bosman MJ, Boecker DR. Selective serotonin reuptake inhibitors: their effect on high-intensity exercise performance. Arch Phys Med Rehabil 2001;82:867–71.
39. Meeusen R, Piacentini MF, van Den Eynde S, et al. Exercise performance is not influenced by a 5-HT reuptake inhibitor. Int J Sports Med 2001;22:329–36.
40. Hildebrand KM, Johnson DJ, Bogle K. Comparison of patterns of alcohol use between high school and college athletes and nonathletes. Coll Student J 2001;35:358–65.
41. Green GA, Uryasz FD, Petr TA, et al. NCAA study of substance use and abuse habits of college student–athletes. Clin J Sport Med 2001;11:51–6.
42. Ford JA. Substance use among college athletes: a comparison based on sport/team affiliation. J Am Coll Health 2007;55(6):367–73.
43. Tricker R. Painkilling drugs in collegiate athletics: knowledge, attitudes, and use of student athletes. J Drug Educ 2000;30:313–24.
44. Pope HG, Katz DL. Affective and psychotic symptoms associated with anabolic steroids use. Am J Psychiatry 1988;145:487–90.
45. McCabe SE, Brower KJ, West BT, et al. Trends in nonmedical use of anabolic steroids by US college students: results from four national surveys. Drug Alcohol Depend 2007;90:243–51.
46. Tricker R, Connolly D. Drugs and the college athlete: an analysis of the attitudes of student athletes at risk. J Drug Educ 1997;27:105–19.
47. Pope HG, Katz DL. Psychiatric and medical effects of anabolic–androgenic steroid use: a controlled study of 160 athletes. Arch Gen Psychiatry 1994;51:375–82.
48. Moser RS. The growing public health concern of sports concussion: the new psychology practice frontier. Prof Psychol Res Pr 2007;38(6):699–704.
49. Broshek DK, Barth JT. Neuropsychological assessment of the amateur athlete. In: Bailes J, Day A, editors. Neurological sports medicine: a guide for physicians and athletic trainers. Rolling Meadows (IL): The American Association of Neurological Surgeons; 2001. p. 155–68.
50. Freeman JR, Barth JT, Broshek DK, et al. Sports injuries. In: Silver JM, McAllister TW, Yudofsky SC, editors. Textbook of traumatic brain injury. Washington, DC: American Psychiatric Publishing; 2005. p. 453–76.

51. Erlanger D, Feldman D, Kutner K, et al. Development and validation of a Web-based neuropsychological test protocol for sports-related return-to-play decision making. Arch Clin Neuropsychol 2003;18:293–316.
52. Erlanger D, Kaushik T, Cantu R, et al. Symptom-based assessment of concussion severity. J Neurosurg 2003;98:477–84.
53. Conn JM, Annest JL, Gilchrist J. Sports and recreation-related injury episodes in the US population, 1997–1999. Inj Prev 2003;9:117–23.
54. Centers for Disease Control and Prevention (CDC). Sports-related injuries among high school athletes in the United States, 2005–06 school year. MMWR Morb Mortal Wkly Rep 2006;55(38):1037–40.
55. Brewer BW, Petrie TA. Psychopathology in sport and excercise. In: Van Raalte JL, Brewer BW, editors. Explorign sport and excercise psychology. 2nd edition. Washington, DC: American Psychological Association; 2001. p. 307–23.
56. Rotella RJ, Heyman SR. Stress, injury and the psychological rehabilitation of athletes. In: Willams JM, editor. Applied sports psychology: personal growth to peak performance. Palo Alto (CA): Mayfield; 1986. p. 343–64.
57. Kubler-Ross E. On death and dying. London: McMillan; 1969.
58. Leddy MH, Lambert MJ, Ogles BM. Psychological consequences of athletic injury among high-level competitors. Res Q Exerc Sport 1994;65:347–54.
59. Junge A. The influence of psychological factors on sports injuries. Am J Sports Med 2000;28:10–5.
60. Williams JM, Andersen MB. Psychosocial antecedents of sport injury and inter-ventions for risk reduction. In: Eklund RC, Tenenbaum G, editors. Handbook of sport psychology. Hoboken (NJ): John Wiley & Sons, Inc; 2007. p. 379–403.
61. Johnson U, Ivarsson A. Psychological predictors of sport injuries among junior soccer players. Scand J Med Sci Sports 2011;21(1):129–36.
62. Gould D, Udry E, Bridges D, et al. Coping with season-ending injuries. Sport Psychol 1997;11:379–99.
63. Prentice WE. The athletic trainer. In: Mueller FO, Ryan AJ, editors. Prevention of athletic injuries: the role of the sports medicine team. Philadelphia: FA Davis; 1991. p. 101–13.
64. Begel D. Psychotherapy with the performing athlete. In: Begel D, Burton R, editors. Sport psychiatry: theory and practice. New York: WW Norton; 2000. p. 191–205.

The Athlete's Pharmacy

Mario Ciocca, MD[a],*, Harry Stafford, MD[a], Ronnie Laney, MD[b]

KEYWORDS

• Medication • Athlete • Pharmacy

Athletes use a variety of substances for the treatment of pain, injury, common illnesses, or to gain an advantage in competition. These substances include prescription medications, over-the-counter medications, nonregulated supplements and, in some instances, illegal or banned substances. A growing concern is that many young athletes may use potentially dangerous, but legal, medications without consulting health professionals. In addition, the combination of these medications with other over-the-counter medications or supplements may lead to a greater risk of side effects. Physicians providing care for athletes should be aware of any medications that an athlete is taking and how these substances may interact with performance, exercise, environment, and other medicines. Moreover, it is vital that physicians are familiar with these medications so that athletes are properly educated on the potential benefits and/or risks and how each substance may affect the body.

MEDICATION CHOICE

Athletes are subject to the same illnesses and injuries as nonathletes. Not surprisingly, the use of over-the-counter medications by athletes is a growing problem. Common medications used by athletes either for self-treatment or as prescribed by a health professional may have unexpected health consequences. The physician should always be aware of whether the drug is absolutely needed or if better alternatives exist. In addition, the physician will need to consider multiple issues that may not be considered in the nonathlete. Thought must be given to such issues as: Are there side effects that may be distressing to the athlete such as diarrhea? Are there side effects that may be exacerbated by exercise such as dehydration? Are there effects that in combination with exercise may bring an undesired effect? Is the medicine going to affect proper physiologic response to exercise? Finally, the physician needs to be

---

The authors have no funding or disclosures.
a James A Taylor Campus Health Service, UNC Sports Medicine, University of North Carolina, CB#7470, Chapel Hill, NC 27599, USA
b Department of Family Medicine, University of North Carolina, 590 Manning Drive, Chapel Hill, NC 27599, USA
* Corresponding author.
E-mail address: ciocca@email.unc.edu

Clin Sports Med 30 (2011) 629–639
doi:10.1016/j.csm.2011.03.003
0278-5919/11/$ – see front matter © 2011 Elsevier Inc. All rights reserved.

familiar with the organization under whose rules the athlete is competing and the medications that are prohibited.

NONSTEROIDAL ANTI-INFLAMMATORY DRUGS

Due to the physical rigors of practice and sport competition, athletes of all types are subject to pain and injury. Nonsteroidal anti-inflammatory drugs (NSAIDs) are among the most common classes of drugs used to treat pain and injury. According to some estimates, there were approximately 85 million prescriptions for NSAIDs written in 2002, totaling $3 billion. If over-the-counter medications were included, the total increases substantially to almost $30 billion.[1] One survey of 604 high school football players found that 75% had used NSAIDs within the prior 3 months, and 15% considered themselves daily users.[2]

Some common NSAID forms are ibuprofen, naproxen, diclofenac, ketorolac, and aspirin. NSAIDs work primarily by blocking the enzyme cyclooxygenase (COX). COX converts arachidonic acid into prostaglandins and thromboxane. Prostaglandins are involved in the production of pain, inflammation, and fever. Prostaglandins are also involved in the protection of gastric mucosa; therefore, blockade of this pathway leads to the gastrointestinal (GI) side effects seen with NSAID use[2] including gastritis, ulcer disease, and GI bleeding. Thromboxane is involved in platelet aggregation; blockade of this pathway leads to an increased risk of bleeding in at-risk patients.[2]

Many undesirable side effects have been documented from the use of NSAIDs. Most of these involve the GI system, for example, ulcers or bleeding. Proton pump inhibitors have been shown to reduce the frequency and severity of GI symptoms in those at risk. Cardiovascular effects include risk of stroke, myocardial infarction, and thrombotic events.[1] Fortunately, most athletes are young and healthy and thus unlikely to experience many of the cardiovascular effects. Renal toxicity is fortunately rare, but analgesic nephropathy with reversible renal toxicity has been documented in adolescents. This finding is of particular concern because many adolescents are not aware of the potential danger of some of these medications, as evidenced by 63% of surveyed adolescents not considering aspirin potentially harmful.[2] Furthermore, up to 76% had used medications without consulting a health care professional.[2] NSAID use may lead to decreased renal perfusion, and can exacerbate renal insufficiency caused by certain situations such as dehydration. Another concern with NSAID use, especially in endurance athletes, is the potential to cause or exacerbate exercise-associated hyponatremia. The primary etiology may be a reduction in glomerular filtration rate.[1] Symptoms might include nausea, vomiting, lightheadedness, lethargy, and cramps. The physician should therefore be well informed and educate the athlete about other predisposing factors such as overhydration, type of fluid consumed (hypotonic solutions), fluid losses through sweat, and inappropriate elevation of anti-diuretic hormone (vasopressin) through exercise.

NSAIDs are potentially beneficial for short-term recovery of muscle function, and may reduce soreness following exercise.[3] With deep muscle contusions, NSAIDs may decrease edema, and have an analgesic effect allowing quicker recovery of motion.[4] NSAIDs given for at least 2 weeks for muscle contusions may decrease the rate of heterotopic ossification.[4]

While evidence clearly shows that early use of NSAIDs provides pain relief, reduction of inflammation, and earlier return to play, more studies are needed on long-term use.[2] Two animal models showed that piroxicam improved contractile strength and maximal failure force early after injury, but slowed collagen deposition and muscle regeneration.[2] Thus, NSAID use may be appropriate during the acute phase of injury when the inflammatory response is associated with pain, edema, and cell death, but use may be contraindicated in the later stages when regeneration has begun.[5]

Athletes not only use oral NSAIDs but now are starting to use topical NSAIDs. These agents have been available in Europe for some time, and are now available in the United States as diclofenac gel (trade name Voltaren)[1] and topical patch (Flector),[2] although other topical NSAIDs can be formulated through compounding pharmacies. Benefits of topical delivery include a decrease in the adverse effects on gastric mucosa, kidneys, and vascular endothelium, a decreased serum concentration, and fewer drug interactions.[1] Topical NSAIDs have been shown to be effective for treatment of acute painful conditions including sprains, strains, and contusions.[6] In osteoarthritis, topical NSAIDs have been shown to have equal efficacy to oral NSAIDs without the adverse effects.[6] The most common adverse effect is rash or pruritus at the application site, and this may be dependent on the vehicle for delivery.[6]

ASTHMA MEDICATIONS

Asthma is a chronic inflammatory condition of the airways that is characterized by increased pulmonary responsiveness to various stimuli. Clinical symptoms include cough, dyspnea, and wheezing. Athletes may have chronic asthma or purely exercise-induced bronchospasm (EIB). In general, both are more prevalent in competitive and elite athletes when compared with the general population.[7] Estimates range anywhere from 10% of athletes having EIB, with the highest estimate of 45% among cyclists, to 22% of American and Italian athletes suffering from asthma during the previous 3 Olympic Games.[7] The prevalence tends to differ by sport, with some of the highest in cross-country skiers, cold-weather sports, summer endurance sports, and swimmers.[7] There has also been an increase in use of inhaled β-agonists since the 1984 Olympic Games.[7] Whether this increase is due to an increase in disease prevalence or to the purported performance-enhancing effects of these agents remains a topic of debate.

Athletes with EIB should have associated asthma controlled as needed. Short-acting β-agonists are usually used prior to exercise in athletes with EIB. There is some evidence as well for long-acting β-agonists in EIB, with formoterol demonstrating a protective effect.[7] Other medications used include leukotriene receptor antagonists (montelukast, zafirlukast), which can attenuate EIB in 50% of patients.[8] The mast cell stabilizer cromolyn sodium, taken shortly before exercise, is beneficial but not as effective as the short-acting β-agonists.[8] Long-acting β-agonists can be used for EIB or maintenance of asthma, but should not be used alone.[8] The most common adverse effects of β-agonists that have an impact on performance include tachycardia, muscle tremor, headache, and irritability.

Although some of the literature is conflicting, with 2 small studies showing an improvement in performance, most studies fail to show that inhaled β-agonists have any effect on Vo_{2max}, anaerobic threshold, or strength performance.[7] One frequently cited study by Signorile observed an increase in peak performance after inhaled short-acting β-agonists, but this was in recreational athletes and not competitive or elite athletes.[7] It is also unclear whether this was due to any ergogenic effects or just better control of asthma. Ergogenic effects with resultant improvement in strength, performance, and anaerobic power have been seen with oral (but not inhaled) administration of salbutamol. Most studies conclude that there is no ergogenic effect achieved with inhaled β-agonists at therapeutic doses, and thus they are not included on the World Anti-Doping Agency (WADA) list.[7] As of this writing, inhaled preparations of salbutamol and salmeterol no longer need therapeutic use exemptions (TUE), only a declaration of use.[7] The inhaled preparations of formoterol and terbutaline still require TUE. All asthmatic athletes still require documented proof of a diagnosis of asthma, including pulmonary function tests. Those with only EIB require exercise challenge testing.

ALLERGIC RHINITIS

Allergic rhinitis is a very common disease, and can present challenges and concerns to the athlete and medical provider. Ventilation increases during athletic activity, with ultimate transition to a combination of mouth and nose breathing. This process leads to increased inhalation of allergens and particles into the lower airways of the athlete.[9] Also, various sports or environments can increase exposure, exacerbating the problem, such as with swimmers, cold air in winter sports, or in summer and outdoor athletics.[9] Chronic nasal swelling can be associated with snoring, decreased sleep, and fatigue, and thus affect athletic performance. Another challenge is that there are many over-the-counter preparations for allergic diseases, so many athletes may self-treat. Others may just avoid treatment altogether.

Identifying athletes with allergic rhinitis and providing treatment may maximize performance. Optimal treatment would include avoidance of allergens and first-line use of intranasal glucocorticoids.[9] Additional agents may include oral or topical decongestants and newer-generation antihistamines (such as loratidine, fexofenadine, and cetirizine). Immunotherapy, typically via desensitization shots, is an option as well.

ANTIBIOTICS

Antibiotics are commonly used to treat respiratory, skin, or urinary tract infections. Common concerns when choosing an antibiotic include the side effect profile as well as the dosing regimen. Avoidance of antibiotics when use is not justified, choosing one with proper coverage but a lower side effect profile, and ensuring compliance with a simplified dosing regimen all play a part in prescribing for athletes.

Overall, antibiotics are tolerated well, and are not banned or prohibited by any regulatory organization. Penicillins and cephalosporins present no real concern except perhaps for the prevalence of penicillin allergies. Fluoroquinolones, represented most commonly by ciprofloxacin, are approved for use in many infections that may affect the athlete or active patient, such as urinary tract infections, respiratory infections, gastrointestinal infections, and some skin infections. Also, it is the only fluoroquinolone approved for use in certain bone and joint infections.[10] Fluoroquinolones should be used with caution, however. For the athlete and sports medicine provider, a major concern is the risk of tendon injury associated with the use of fluoroquinolones. One study looked at the risk of tendinitis and tendon injury with the use of fluoroquinolones, and determined that use increased the overall risk of tendon injury, with an odds ratio (OR) of 1.4.[11] Tendon rupture was associated with an OR of 1.3, with Achilles tendon rupture having an OR of 4.1.[11] The risk further increased with concomitant use of steroids. The cause of fluoroquinolone-induced tendon injury is not fully known. Other adverse side effects associated with fluoroquinolone use are QT prolongation, poor glycemic control, and phototoxicity.[11]

Over the last two decades, community-acquired methicillin-resistant *Staphylococcus aureus* (CA-MRSA) has emerged as a major community pathogen, and may be seen more frequently in athletes. Once thought to be a nosocomial pathogen only, the community form can infect children and young, otherwise healthy adults.[12] *S aureus* is a commonly occurring organism in skin flora, and thus has a predilection for skin and soft tissue.[12] Its implication in athletics is important because of skin trauma associated with turf burns, abrasions, shaving, and chafing.[12] The problem is exacerbated by the sharing of towels, equipment, close quarters (training rooms, showers), and prolonged contact during sport.[12,13] When an athlete or affected individual does require antibiotic treatment, trimethoprim-sulfamethoxazole, doxycycline, or clindamycin are appropriate first-line choices. Cultures should be performed to confirm sensitivity. Clindamycin is a common choice, but is associated with diarrhea and risk of *Clostridium difficile* colitis.[12] Other treatment options being considered are decolonization, or eradication, with various soap baths. The literature is not clear as to the optimal method for decolonization. One method involves using topical mupirocin, twice daily, intranasally. As with other topical preparations, there is a reduction in toxicity and effects sometimes associated with systemic absorption. However, the efficacy of mupirocin monotherapy remains unclear, and there have been reports of growing resistance.[12]

ACNE

Acne is a common skin problem among adolescents and young athletes. In athletes the acne may also occur or be exacerbated by certain equipment that is worn. Often it is primarily a social or cosmetic concern. Nevertheless, it is important that acne be addressed because many of the medications used to treat this condition can affect the health of the athlete, or have significant side effects that warrant consideration of the necessity of use. Two initial treatment choices are topical antibiotics and benzoyl peroxide, usually used in combination to reduce the emergence of resistance.[14] Topical clindamycin and erythromycin are 2 of the most widely used antibiotics in gel or cream form. Topical tetracyclines are used less often.[14]

Topical antibiotics have been shown to work through both anti-inflammatory and antimicrobial mechanisms. The anti-inflammatory effects are not fully understood, but are thought to be caused by several different mechanisms. Current hypotheses suggest a reduction in leukocyte chemotaxis and other chemotactic factors, reduction in free fatty acids at the skin surface due to reduction in lipase production by *Propionibacterium acnes*, and reduction in the burden of *P acnes*.[14] More research is needed, but it is thought that the benefit of antibiotics in acne is due more to the anti-inflammatory mechanism than reduction in the number of bacteria.[14] This proposal is further supported by the fact that *P acnes* is not truly pathogenic, and acne is thought to be more likely a function of the host inflammatory response.[15] Topical antibiotics are generally well tolerated, with the main effects being local irritation, erythema, itching, peeling, dryness, and burning. Their favorable profile also makes them good choices for use in summer, when athletes are generally more active outdoors.[14] Resistance may develop, especially with monotherapy, which is why these therapies are often used in combination with benzoyl peroxide.[15]

Benzoyl peroxide acts as a powerful antimicrobial agent, and has been shown to be as effective as topical antibiotics but without risk of resistance.[14] Some concerns associated with its use are cutaneous irritation and dryness, and bleaching of hair, clothes, and linens. However, most of these occur in the first few days of treatment and subside with continued use.[14] Benzoyl peroxide exerts its anti-inflammatory effect by inhibiting reactive oxygen species in neutrophils, though the exact mechanism is unknown.[14]

The retinoids continue to be a mainstay of severe and nodulocystic acne.[16] However, these drugs continue to be used with caution, given their rather severe adverse effects. Retinoids have been shown to be teratogenic, and reproductive-aged females taking the drug must undergo monthly pregnancy tests and are monitored through a federally mandated registry program.[17] Of concern for athletes are reports of back pain and joint aches as well as elevated creatine kinase levels with use of this medication.[16,18]

Oral antibiotics are widely used in acne but are not without potential complications. In particular, the tetracyclines are well known to cause phototoxic cutaneous reactions. The incidence of these reactions has been reported to be around 5%. A study of 106 acne patients found a much higher incidence (35.8%) and suggested that the phenomenon is dose related; 20% of patients taking 150 mg/d of doxycycline developed a light-sensitive rash, whereas 42% of those taking 200 mg/d were affected.[19] For those taking minocycline, medication side effects must be kept in the differential for athlete complaints of joint pain. Minocycline may also be associated with a lupus-like illness with joint pain, myalgias, and fever.[20] The tetracyclines are also associated with a significant risk for pill esophagitis.

ORAL CONTRACEPTIVES

Female athletes use oral contraception for various reasons. In addition to their use for birth control, oral contraceptives may be useful in controlling dysmenorrhea and reducing the symptoms of menstruation, thus reducing time lost from participation by controlling symptoms such as severe cramps. Manipulation of oral contraceptives can be used to the female athlete's advantage for athletic events by skipping the placebo pills and continuing the active pills, to prolong the interval between menstrual periods.

The female athlete triad is a combination of disordered eating, menstrual irregularities, and osteopenia/osteoporosis. Early recognition and management assists in the prevention of acute or long-term problems.[21] Correcting the low estrogen status of these athletes is of primary importance, particularly for bone metabolism. Oral contraceptives are the therapy of choice for known deficiencies. Evidence is still too controversial, or simply inadequate, to support routine estrogen supplementation for the prevention of stress fractures or improvement in bone health.[22]

Side effects that often concern the athlete include headaches, nausea, fluid retention, and weight gain. There is also an increased risk of deep venous thrombosis. A few studies have found a decrease in Vo_{2max} among trained female athletes on oral contraceptives.[23] The effect of oral contraceptives on ligaments is conflicting, and more research is needed.[24,25]

ANTIDEPRESSANTS/ANXIOLYTICS/STIMULANTS

The use of antidepressants and other psychoactive drugs, particularly stimulants, has increased dramatically among children and adolescents over the last two decades, with an estimated 1.4 million Americans younger than 18 years receiving antidepressant prescriptions in 2002.[26] The introduction of the selective serotonin reuptake inhibitors (SSRIs) made antidepressant therapy far more feasible in athletes because of their favorable side effect profile.[26] A logical first choice has often been fluoxetine (Prozac), with its approved use in younger patients and minimal effects on weight.[26] Many such agents are now available and widely used. In addition to pharmacotherapy, evidence supports a multimodal approach that includes psychotherapy.[26] Use of antidepressants always carries an increased risk of suicidal thoughts and behaviors. Such behavior does occur, but is rare, and the general consensus favors the use of SSRIs in light of the overall reduction in actual suicides.[26]

The diagnosis of attention-deficit/hyperactivity disorder (ADHD) among children and adolescents continues to increase as well, with stimulant use doubling every 4 to 7 years.[27] Clinical manifestations are characterized by two main symptom complexes: poor ability to focus and maintain attention, and impulsivity and hyperactivity.[27] Also, more than half of those children with ADHD carry one or more comorbid conditions such as learning disability, poor motor function, depression, anxiety, and personality disorders.[27] Athletes may derive unfair benefits in improved concentration and coordination, and stimulants are thus prohibited by the International Olympic Committee.[27] At present, the WADA Code also prohibits stimulant use. Athletic concerns with the use of stimulants include vasoconstriction in the skin, increased blood pressure, and decreased thermoregulation. Caution should be used when athletes are participating in hot conditions or if they are prone to dehydration. The potential cardiac effects should also be monitored. Physicians must be aware that athletes may be unknowingly taking other stimulants in supplements or decongestants. Athletes must also be monitored to ensure that they are prescribed the correct dosage to prevent insomnia and weight loss due to appetite suppression.[28]

CARDIOVASCULAR MEDICATIONS

Diuretics and β-blockers are drugs that may be effective in treating hypertension, but should be used with caution in athletes. Because diuretics act on the kidneys to reduce plasma volume, the resultant risk of dehydration may affect performance.[29] Other potential concerns may involve rapid and reversible shifts in weight, especially in sports where weight plays a major role such as boxing, gymnastics, wrestling, or swimming. The athletic staff must also monitor kidney function and electrolytes, as dehydration and hypokalemia may be exacerbated from exercising in the heat. Diuretics are also banned by many organizations because of their possible use as masking agents for illicit substances.

β-Blockers are a class of cardiovascular medications used for hypertension as well as anxiety or essential tremor. These drugs are banned in specific precision sports such as rifle shooting and archery.[30] β-Blockers may adversely affect performance in the athlete via a decrease in Vo_{2max}, a decrease in cardiac output, and alterations in fuel use, thermoregulation, and skeletal muscle recruitment patterns.[30] In addition, there is an increase in perceived exertion during prolonged submaximal exercise, and they may also exacerbate underlying asthma.[30] If this category is used, then a selective β-blocker is a better choice than the nonselective β-blockers.

Because of the problems with β-blockers and diuretics, angiotensin-converting enzyme (ACE) inhibitors, angiotensin II receptor blockers, or calcium channel blockers may be more appropriate first-line therapies in the athlete with high blood pressure. ACE inhibitors and angiotensin II receptor blockers do not alter the heart rate response or exercise tolerance during submaximal exercise.[30] Calcium channel blockers can have a variable effect on exercise heart rate, but exercise tolerance is usually unaffected.[30]

Another category of medication of concern in athletes is the statin family, used for hypercholesterolemia. Treatment guidelines are clear for hyperlipidemia.

Therapeutic lifestyle changes are first-line with reductions in weight, dietary changes, and increase in exercise. If the use of a statin is indicated, the main concern is the effect on muscle. Myalgias and elevated liver enzymes are common side effects.[31] The most serious complication, fatal rhabdomyolysis, is rare and estimated to occur once per 10 million prescriptions.[31] If this is recognized early enough, prompt discontinuation may lead to prevention of this serious complication.[31]

DOPING CONTROL

Performance enhancement during competition has been known since ancient times. As early as 776 AD, the early Olympians were using substances such as mushrooms, figs, and strychnine to compete at an advantage.[32] Today, athletes are subject to monitoring for the use of performance enhancers at each level of competition, and physicians must be aware of this process and the rules that athletes at each level must follow.

At the international level, WADA was started to organize the Anti-Doping Program and to harmonize antidoping policies and regulations within sport organizations and among governments. WADA was established in 1999 as an international independent agency, composed and funded equally by the sport movement and governments of the world. Its key activities include scientific research, education, development of anti-doping capacities, and monitoring of the World Anti-Doping Code.[33]

At the national level in the United States, the US Anti-Doping Agency was started in 2000 as a nonprofit, nongovernmental agency for Olympic, Pan American, and Paralympic sports. Its purpose is to preserve sport through research, education, and enforcement and regulation. It also provides research to better detect illicit substances in an attempt to truly sanction only the guilty athletes trying to gain an unfair advantage over those competing "clean." Another purpose is to educate athletes, coaches, students, parents, scientists, government, official organizations, and health professionals regarding the practice of doping and the various measures of doping control.

Many professional sports have their own antidoping organizations. Their policies, testing, and punishments vary among the sports. At the collegiate level, doping is monitored by the National Collegiate Athletic Association (NCAA).

PROHIBITED MEDICATIONS

As a prescribing physician, it is important to know whether an athlete is monitored by an antidoping organization. Avoidance of prohibited medications will save the athlete from potential penalties or sanctions. There are many common medications that may be prohibited. One common medication is β-agonist therapy used for asthma. There is some evidence that this class may be performance enhancing, and there is concern about excessive and inappropriate use. The NCAA does permit β2-agonists via inhalation. WADA, however, only permits inhalation with salbutamol/albuterol and salmeterol, and one must not exceed 1600 μg/d of salbutamol.

Care needs to be taken with prescription of diuretics for the treatment of hypertension or polycystic ovarian disease. Both the NCAA and WADA ban diuretics because of their potential use as masking agents for drug tests. Stimulants are another class that may be widely used whether prescribed for attention-deficit disorder, narcolepsy, or weight loss, or more commonly taken over the counter as a decongestant. WADA bans in-competition use of amphetamine and amphetamine-derivative medications. Pseudoephedrine was previously banned and then placed onto the WADA monitoring system. There has been an increase in use and abuse as well as some evidence for performance-enhancing effect; therefore, pseudoephedrine is currently banned at a urinary level of 150 μg/mL or above, which may be reached with a daily dose of 240 mg. The NCAA does not ban pseudoephedrine.

Glucocorticoids are not prohibited by the NCAA but are banned by WADA for in-competition use when administered orally, intravenously, or intramuscularly. Nasal steroids are not banned, and steroids via inhalation simply require a declaration of use. Some medications are not completely prohibited but are limited in certain sports because of their mechanism of action. β-Blockers fall into this category because of their curtailment of unwanted tremor or hand motion. The recent increased use of platelet-rich plasma (PRP) in tendon injury has also brought attention to this method as a possible performance enhancer. At present, PRP is banned by WADA for direct injection into muscle but is permitted for injection directly into tendons.[33]

THERAPEUTIC USE EXEMPTION/DECLARATION OF USE

An athlete may be able to take a medication banned by WADA by filing a TUE at least 30 days prior to competition. Certain criteria are required to obtain approval for a TUE, and can be used for acute or chronic conditions. First, that the athlete's health would be significantly affected if the drug were withheld. In addition, that there is no improvement in performance other than what would be expected from returning to normal health. Third, that there is no reasonable alternative to the banned drug the athlete is seeking to use. Finally, the drug is not being used as a result of a condition that was caused by taking a prohibited substance. Applications for TUE are kept confidential, and include a comprehensive medical history and results of all examinations, laboratory tests, and imaging studies. There also must be a physician statement substantiating the need for the drug and the lack of an alternative.[34]

SUMMARY

Clinicians involved in the care of athletes need to be aware of multiple issues before prescribing medications. There needs to be diligence in prescribing medications only when appropriate, and in staying abreast of other medications and supplements that may interact with the new medication. An athlete will not tolerate adverse effects on performance, and there needs to be an awareness of medications that may physiologically affect performance or cause side effects that may hinder athletes' physical abilities. Finally, the clinician needs to be aware of governing antidoping bodies, and avoid prescribing medications that will lead to harmful penalties or disqualification. The team physician who is cognizant of all of these factors will optimize care of the athlete.

REFERENCES

1. Madden CC, Putukian M, Young CC, et al. Sports pharmacology of pain and inflammation control in athletes. Netter's sports medicine. Philadelphia: Saunders, Elsevier; 2010. p. 47–51, 171–83.
2. Feucht CL, Patel DR. Analgesics and anti-inflammatory medications in sports: use and abuse. Pediatr Clin North Am 2010;57:751–74.
3. Lanier AB. Use of nonsteroidal anti-inflammatory drugs following exercise induced muscle injury. Sports Med 2003;33(3):177–86.
4. Larson CM, Almekinders LC, Karas SG, et al. Evaluating and managing muscle contusions and myositis ossificans. Phys Sportsmed 2002;30(2):41–6.
5. Paoloni JA, Milne C, Orchard J, et al. Non-steroidal anti-inflammatory drugs in sports medicine: guidelines for practical but sensible use. Br J Sports Med 2009;43:863–5.
6. Haroutiunian S, Drennan DA, Lipman AG. Topical NSAID therapy for musculoskeletal pain. Pain Med 2010;11:535–49.
7. Wolfarth B, Wuestenfeld JC, Kindermann W. Ergogenic effects of inhaled B2-agonists in non-asthmatic athletes. Endocrinol Metab Clin North Am 2010; 39:75–87.

8. National Asthma Education and Prevention Program. Expert Panel Report 3 (EPR-3): guidelines for the diagnosis and management of asthma—summary report 2007. J Allergy Clin Immunol 2007;120(5):S94–138.

9. Alaranta A, Alaranta H, Heliovaara M, et al. Allergic rhinitis and pharmacological management in elite athletes. Med Sci Sports Exerc 2005;35(5):707–11.

10. Bolon M. The newer fluoroquinolones. Infect Dis Clin North Am 2009;23:1027–51.

11. Corrao G, Zambon A, Bertù L, et al. Evidence of tendinitis provoked by fluoroquinolone treatment: a case-controlled study. Drug Saf 2006;29:889–96.

12. Romano R, Lu D, Holtom P. Outbreak of community-acquired methicillin resistant Staphylococcus aureus skin infections among a collegiate football team. J Athl Train 2006;41(2):141–5.

13. Rakel R. Textbook of family medicine. 7th edition. Philadelphia: Saunders Elsevier; 2007.

14. Dreno B. Topical antibacterial therapy for acne vulgaris. Drugs 2004;64(21): 2389–97.

15. Leyden JJ, Del Rosso JQ, Webster GF. Clinical considerations in the treatment of acne vulgaris and other inflammatory skin disorders: a status report. Dermatol Clin 2009;27:1–15.

16. Landau M, Mesterman R, Ophir J, et al. Clinical significance of markedly elevated serum creatine kinase levels in patients with acne on isotretinoin. Acta Derm Venereol 2001;81:350–2.

17. Clarke SB, Nelson AM, George RE, et al. Pharmacologic modulation of sebaceous gland activity: mechanisms and clinical applications. Dermatol Clin 2007;25:137–46.

18. Jah MM. Hip pain and retinoids (isotretinoin). Pak J Med Sci 2011;27(1):196–8.

19. Yong CK, Prendiville J, Peacock DL, et al. An unusual presentation of doxycycline-induced photosensitivity. Pediatrics 2000;106:e13.

20. Elkayam O, Levartovsky D, Brautbar C, et al. Clinical and immunological study of 7 patients with minocycline-induced autoimmune phenomena. Am J Med 1998; 105(6):484–7.

21. Ray T. Female athletes: medical concerns. Athl Ther Today 2005;40(1):40–1.

22. Beals KA, Meyer NL. Female athlete triad update. Clin Sports Med 2007;26: 69–89.

23. Rechechi C, Dawson B, Goodman C. Athletic performance and the oral contraceptive. Int J Sports Physiol Perform 2009;4:151–62.

24. Martineau PA, Al-Jassir F, Lenczner E, et al. Effect of oral contraceptive pill on ligamentous laxity. Clin J Sport Med 2004;14:281–6.

25. Hicks-Little CA, Thatcher JR, Hauth JM, et al. Menstrual cycle stage and oral contraceptive effects on anterior tibial displacement in collegiate female athletes. J Sports Med Phys Fitness 2007;47(2):255–60.

26. Calles J. Depression in children and adolescents. Prim Care 2007;34:243–58.

27. Hickey G, Fricker P. Attention deficit hyperactivity disorder, CNS stimulants, and sport. Sports Med 1999;1:11–21.

28. Bouchard R, Weber AR, Geiger JD. Informed decision-making on sympathomimetic use in sport and health. Clin J Sport Med 2002;12:209–24.

29. Fagard R. Athletes with systemic hypertension. Cardiol Clin 2007;25:441–8.

30. Derman W. FIMS position statement—antihypertensive medications and exercise. Int J Sports Med 2008;9(1):32–8.

31. Reamy B, Thompson P. Lipid disorders in athletes. Curr Sports Med Rep 2004;3: 70–6.

32. Pommering T. Erythropoietin and other blood-boosting methods. Pediatr Clin North Am 2007;54:691–9.
33. The World Anti-Doping Code. The 2010 Prohibited List International Standard. WADA website.
34. World Anti-Doping Programme. Therapeutic use exemption guidelines. Version 4. 2010. WADA website.

The International Athlete—Advances in Management of Jet Lag Disorder and Anti-Doping Policy

Daniel Herman, MD, PhD[a], John M. MacKnight, MD[b],
Amy E. Stromwall, MD[c,d], Dilaawar J. Mistry, MD, ATC[e,*]

KEYWORDS

- International athlete • Jet lag (JL) • Sleep aids
- Anti-doping policy

International athletic competitions continue to evolve rapidly on a global scale, both in the frequency of competitions and the potential financial benefits for athletes. As a result, the "modern," "high-performance," "international athlete" is subject to frequent travel across several "time zones" on a regular basis. The implications of significant monetary gains and losses serve as an impetus for the international athlete to maximize rest during long travel, and expeditiously overcome the detrimental effects of "jet lag" (JL), so as to perform at the highest level of international competition worldwide. As a result, athletes frequently use various medications to ensure both adequate rest and expedite recovery after tedious flights. Within the context of "permissible medication" use by the international athlete, strict compliance with

There was no funding needed to support this work.
The authors have no financial disclosure.
[a] Department of Physical Medicine and Rehabilitation, University of Virginia Health System, 545 Ray C. Hunt Drive, Charlottesville, VA 22908-1004, USA
[b] Department of Medicine, University of Virginia Health System, 415 Ray C. Hunt Drive, Suite 2100, Charlottesville, VA 22908-0671, USA
[c] Summit Orthopedics Ltd, 310 Smith Avenue North, St Paul, MN 55102, USA
[d] Departments of Athletics and Physical Medicine and Rehabilitation, University of Virginia Health System, 545 Ray C. Hunt Drive, Suite 240, PO Box 801004, Charlottesville, VA 22908-1004, USA
[e] U.S.A. Swimming, 1 Olympic Plaza, Colorado Springs, CO 80909, USA
* Corresponding author. Department of Physical Medicine and Rehabilitation, University of Virginia Health System, PO Box 801004, 545 Ray C. Hunt Drive, Suite 240, Charlottesville, VA 22908-1004.
E-mail address: DM5F@hscmail.mcc.virginia.edu

Clin Sports Med 30 (2011) 641–659
doi:10.1016/j.csm.2011.03.009
0278-5919/11/$ – see front matter © 2011 Elsevier Inc. All rights reserved.

anti-doping policy is pivotal before and during competition. Furthermore, the advent of new medications requires constant vigilance by sports medicine personnel, to both evaluate drug efficacy and judiciously prescribe medications approved by the World Anti-Doping Agency (WADA) and the US Anti-Doping Agency (USADA). The purpose of this article is to provide the reader with an understanding of the physiology of JL, with updates on the effects and management of JL, and with the use of various medications to overcome the potential deleterious effects of JL on peak human performance. Last, recent updates on anti-doping policies are discussed.

JET LAG DISORDER
Introduction

Long-haul travel is often associated with the effects of "travel fatigue," which includes complaints of general malaise, headache, and diminished mood states. Travel fatigue results from stresses related to the act of transportation itself. These include being confined to a cramped environment with little opportunity for physical activity, stressors associated with making travel arrangements, dehydration during flights, and disrupted sleep and dietary habits. Travel fatigue generally rapidly abates within a day after arrival with sufficient rest.

Flight dysrhythmia, commonly known as "jet lag disorder," occurs as a result of rapid desynchronization of normal circadian rhythms ("the body clock") with exogenous time cues, termed *zeitgebers* ("time givers"). This syndrome may occur after transmeridian travel over more than 2 time zones, and involves a constellation of symptoms, including poor sleep characteristics (eg, initiation, maintenance, and quality), reduced task performance (eg, sprint time, concentration, reaction time), and disruption of gastrointestinal function (eg, changes in bowel habits, constipation, appetite changes).

In contrast to travel fatigue, symptoms stemming from JL persist for a number of days and bear a relationship to the number of meridians traversed and the direction traveled. As a general rule, resynchronization occurs over 1.0 to 1.5 days per time zone change, with shorter resynchronization periods associated with westward travel compared with eastward travel.[1] The severity of symptoms increases in general proportion to the number of time zones traveled, and is more troublesome with eastward than westward travel.[2,3] It should also be noted that there is a significant range of variation in resynchronization times across different circadian functions and individuals.

The topic of sleep issues in the athlete was extensively reviewed in an issue of *Clinics in Sports Medicine* in 2005.[4] This article largely focuses on providing updates to the existing evidence and clinical recommendations since the last publication, including the effects of transmeridian travel on athletes, as well as the evidence supporting management options, which includes sleep scheduling, exercise, light-exposure techniques, and the use of pharmacologic aids. Important considerations regarding special athletic populations are discussed. To effectively cover these topics, a brief review of the chronobiology of JL and the effects of transmeridian travel is imperative.

The Chronobiology of Jet Lag

The "central body clock," located in the suprachiasmatic nuclei at the base of the hypothalamus, functions as a result of complex rhythmic genetically mediated activity, with an intrinsic periodicity of slightly longer than 24 hours ("circadian" stems from *circa* meaning about and *dian* meaning day). Its functional periodicity is modulated by several factors, including environmental light via the retinohypothalamic tract and physical activity via the intergeniculate leaflet.[5] Recent evidence suggests that several "peripheral body clocks" may also exert feedback effects on the rhythm of the "central clock."[6–8] The "central clock" mediates the timing of various physiologic circadian rhythms cyclically. These cycles are resistant to change to provide a measure of stability to the rhythms when confronted with temporary conditions, such as a night with episodes of interrupted sleep. However, this resistance to perturbation is the underlying cause for the syndrome of JL, as desirable shifts in these rhythms are slow to evolve after a rapid alteration in daily habits, such as may result from transmeridian travel.

The "central clock" also governs circadian variations in the sleep-wake cycle via changes in core temperature and secretion of melatonin from the pineal gland. Core temperature minimums generally occur around 0400 hours, with rapid increases in core temperature promoting wakefulness, and rapid decreases in core temperature promoting sleepiness.[9] Conversely, melatonin secretion rapidly increases in the evening after the onset of darkness to promote sleep, and then decreases in the morning.

These rhythms are tracked partially by changes in physical and mental performance, which has been shown to vary with core temperature. Relatively low performance is noted near the nadir of daily core temperature and relatively high performance near the peak. Performance parameters range from simple measures of muscle force, power output, and reaction time to more integrative tasks requiring complex motor timing, decision making, and motivation to maintain a sustained effort.[4,10] The differences between these points of high and low performance can be meaningful in a competitive environment. For example, measures of isometric and dynamic strength have been shown to have circadian variation of as much as 6% to 10% of mean values.[11] Significant variations in sport-specific performance have also been demonstrated in a recent study that found a variation of 5.8 seconds between high and low performance points for a 200-m swim trial.[12] Given a mean performance time of 169.5 seconds, this translates into a length difference of approximately 7 m.

Effects of Transmeridian Travel on Performance

Direct data regarding the effects of transmeridian travel on the performance of athletes are scant. Although the results from these studies tend to demonstrate reduced levels of performance after transmeridian travel, a measure of clarity is lacking owing in part to methodological difficulties.[13] As such, most data related to performance in these settings are gleaned from making inferences regarding the effects of sleep deprivation on the circadian rhythms of various aspects of performance such as strength, flexibility, and motor skills,[14] and from studies using laboratory-induced shifts in circadian rhythms.

Prior studies suggest changes in performance depend in part on the type of athletic task used: more short-duration, anaerobic tasks tend to be more resistant to the effects of acute sleep deprivation, whereas tasks that have significant cognitive demands are more susceptible. This has been reinforced by more recent findings. Bullock and colleagues[15] demonstrated minimal effects of an 8-hour phase advance on 30-m sprint time despite objective and subjective physiologic changes, whereas Bambaeichi and colleagues[16] found no adverse effects of partial sleep loss on maximal muscle strength. More robust data exist regarding the performance of nonathletes, such as those in occupational settings such as pilots, day-evening shift workers, and medical personnel.[17] These studies have had similar findings, with errors in judgment and organization being more prominent compared with "short-burst" physical tasks.

Although JL is commonly proposed as a risk factor for athletic injury, even less is known regarding changes in relative injury risk in athletes after travel. The scientific acumen is extrapolated from studies in occupational settings, and demonstrates that there is an increased risk for accidents after sleep deprivation and shift changes.[17] Additional inferences regarding injury risk are made relying on known diurnal variations in flexibility, cognition, and risk of cardiovascular events; however, the evidence is tenuous at best.

Reduced flexibility has long been cited as a risk factor for injury; however, studies regarding the effect of various stretching protocols on injury risk and performance have been decidedly mixed.[18,19] Neurocognitive performance is also a common component included in injury-risk models, but epidemiologic data are lacking. A recent study suggests a relationship between neurocognitive performance and anterior cruciate ligament injury in collegiate athletes[20]; otherwise, the evidence is limited to small studies on injury proneness in adolescents.[21,22] Finally, the risk of cardiovascular events during exercise does not appear to vary significantly throughout the day, despite known diurnal variations in myocardial ischemia, myocardial infarction, and sudden cardiac death.[23]

In summary, direct and indirect evidence suggests that JL induces performance decrements in sport, although the understanding of this relationship is not robust. Nonetheless, it is important to be cognizant of this important consideration during transmeridian travel for training and/or competition, particularly in those sports with high cognitive and fine-motor requirements. In contrast, there is no direct evidence of increased injury risk in these settings, and available indirect evidence is limited or equivocal with no recent significant advances in this area of study. Although it is reasonable to include considerations of sleep and JL in injury models, as has been proposed elsewhere,[24] more meaningful research is needed.

Managing Transmeridian Travel

Management of JL has been an area of increasing interest, and several recent studies have provided additional evidence to help support known and proposed methods that may be used by athletes and the sports medicine team.

Sleep scheduling

Recent studies have been conducted in an attempt to define the most optimal sleep schedule for travel resulting in phase advances and delays. These investigations appear to support a gradual shift in sleep scheduling in 1-hour increments in advance of and after arrival in a new time zone, to effect changes in the circadian clock. Increments larger than 1 hour may be too fast for the circadian clock, and recent studies have not demonstrated any additional benefits.[25] Furthermore, extra aggressive rates of change will result in additional "jarring" circadian misalignment, and may increase the negative effects of JL on characteristics of sleep, such as initiation.[26] In contrast, the use of gradual 1-hour shifts in recent study protocols with and without varying *zeitgebers* produced minimal subjective changes in symptoms associated with JL.[25,27,28] Thus, slow changes in sleep scheduling both before travel and after arrival may accelerate changes in circadian rhythm without introducing undesirable symptoms.

Strategic napping has also been a strategy of interest. The use of a short nap of 20 to 30 minutes may provide significant recuperation without being long enough to affect re-entrainment in the new time zone.[29] Waterhouse and colleagues[30] demonstrated improved cognition and sprint performance in sleep-deprived athletes who were allowed a post-lunch nap of 30 minutes compared with those without a nap. Interestingly, the measures of performance for this study were short-burst anaerobic tasks, which, as previously noted, tend to be more resistant to sleep deprivation and transmeridian travel. Yet, napping resulted in significant performance improvements in some measures. Notably, this study did not include a nonsleep-deprived control condition, which raises the question of the possible performance benefits of an appropriately timed nap in both sleep-deprived and normal conditions.

Exercise
As previously discussed, performance varies during the day. Thus, it would be logical to manipulate training session schedules in an attempt to align performance peaks with the timing of competition after travel. The diurnal variation in activity and performance may also influence other daily rhythms and thus improve synchronization to new time zones. Atkinson and colleagues[31] noted that current evidence is hampered by difficulty in controlling for activity, subject fitness, and confounding *zeitgebers*. However, these studies tend to indicate a role for exercise in mediating phase delays with westward travel.

More recent evidence supports this assertion. Montaruli and colleagues[32] studied the activity and sleep qualities of participants in the New York Marathon after travel from Milan to New York (phase delay of 6 hours). Study cohorts consisted of a group that trained in the day, a group that trained in the night, and a nonparticipative control group. The participants all trained in the morning after arrival. The evening training group demonstrated a greater shift in activity to the morning and less sleep fragmentation, compared with both morning training and control groups. This study was subject to methodological concerns noted by Atkinson and colleagues,[31] and did not directly measure performance or rhythms such as core body temperature or melatonin. However, it does lend some additional credence to the strategy of shifting training schedules before travel to match phase-delayed schedules in the new time zone. Although prior investigations have been equivocal, a recent study in a well-controlled environment indicates that improved phase advances with eastward travel may also be possible via exercise.[33]

Light exposure
Exposure to sufficiently intense light is recognized as a key *zeitgeber* in the re-entrainment of circadian rhythms, and significant effort has been made to determine the most appropriate protocol. Changes in bright light exposure have also been shown to improve measures of performance. Partial re-entrainment with light exposure has been associated with attenuated attention impairments, fatigue, and job performance in shift workers,[34,35] although it should be noted that there is little evidence on the performance effects of bright light exposure in athletes. Timing, intensity, dosing pattern, and wavelength may all be key factors for consideration.

Bright light in the evening and beginning of the sleep phase will produce phase delays, whereas bright light in the morning and end of the sleep phase will produce phase advances. Data regarding precise timing for optimal effects is reflected in the works of Paul and colleagues,[36] who investigated phase shifts under various light exposure timing conditions in individuals with normal sleep times between 2300 and 0700 hours. They demonstrated that bright light exposure within the 0600 and 0700 hours results in the largest phase advances, whereas exposure within the 0200 hour resulted in the largest phase delays among the time periods studied. This precise timing may be impractical depending on circumstances, and significant practical outcomes have been achieved using exposure at similar times.[37,38] Furthermore, control of light exposure at all times may be impractical, particularly on the day of travel and in other circumstances when it is necessary to be outside in natural light. However, light exposure at undesirable times during re-entrainment may be controlled via dark sunglasses, and has been demonstrated to be important for adapting to a night shift in occupational settings.[34,39]

The effects of light intensity and wavelength have also been studied. Positive results have been demonstrated in studies using light visors or light boxes and intensities as low as 3000 lux.[40–42] Nevertheless, it is possible that higher intensities may be required with individuals with higher than average normal daily light exposure.[8] Prior studies indicate that light-mediated circadian rhythms may be most sensitive to shorter blue wavelength light, with exposure to this end of the light spectrum resulting in higher alertness[43,44] and maximal melatonin suppression.[45–47] However, studies thus far indicate that blue-enriched bright light is not superior to white light in promoting phase delays[48] or phase advances.[49]

Melatonin

Use of exogenous melatonin to combat the effects of time shifts has been endorsed by the American Academy of Sleep Medicine,[50] and has additional beneficial qualities that may assist with adjusting to phase changes. Melatonin may simplistically be considered as being "12 hours out of phase" with core body temperature and normal light exposure. Phase delays may thus be affected by administration in late sleep or early morning, and phase advances may be produced by administration in the evening or early sleep period. These phase shifts, after use of both immediate and sustained-release melatonin, have been demonstrated repeatedly,[27,51–53] and have been shown to have additive effects with other strategies such as light exposure.[53] Although wide-ranging and occasionally conflicting results have previously been noted on the effects of melatonin on performance,[54] recent studies have provided some clarity.

There are indications that melatonin ingestion during awake periods results in immediate cognitive performance decrements,[55,56] but has not been shown to adversely affect short duration tasks of strength and power.[57] Furthermore, these decrements in cognitive performance appear to be short-lived, because after sleep interruption and short daytime naps following melatonin ingestion, cognition was shown to be impacted marginally at best.[58,59] Similarly, no decrements in performance have been observed after a full, 8-hour period of rest.[60] Sustained-release forms of melatonin are also commercially available, and may affect cognition for more prolonged periods. However, in a recent study by Paul and colleagues,[52] similar phase advances were observed with rapid-release, sustained-release, and rapid plus sustained-release formulas. Thus, use of rapid-release forms may obviate some of the concern for cognitive decrements with sustained-release forms, while maintaining the benefits of phase changes.

As is the case with any pharmacologic agent, knowledge of its side-effect profile and contraindications is important. A concerning side effect of the use of melatonin in elite athletes is its tendency to cause reductions of blood pressure,[61,62] especially in light of relatively lower blood pressures among athletes. Additionally, melatonin may reduce insulin sensitivity and induce gastrointestinal distress,[63] and may have performance implications in athletes if taken at inappropriate times relative to training and competition. It should also be noted that over-the-counter (OTC) forms of melatonin are considered supplements by the Federal Drug Administration in the United States, and are therefore not subject to the stringent standards of scrutiny for prescription medications. Use of unregulated, contaminated forms of melatonin may result in unintentional exposure of banned substances, and potentially jeopardize the athlete's competitive status.

Melatonin receptor agonists, such as ramelteon, are alternatives to OTC melatonin. These medications have more specific receptor affinity than melatonin, longer half-lives,[64] and appear to be superior to melatonin in promoting sleep initiation and maintenance, particularly when using light exposure appropriately.[51] Akin to melatonin, these agents have demonstrated to be effective in inducing circadian phase shifts.[65,66] Consequently, at first glance, these medications appear to be a promising alternative to melatonin. Yet, it is important to note that the evidence thus far is limited only to the treatment of insomnia, and there are no data regarding its effects on subjects undergoing transmeridian travel or its effects on the performance of athletes, which is a justifiable concern given its longer half-life.

Sleep aids

Impaired sleep is often the most bothersome symptom of JL, and curtailed sleep reduces the response to light in re-entrainment.[67] In addition to the melatonin receptor agonists described previously, several nonbenzodiazepine hypnotics may also be an option for improving sleep after transmeridian travel. Medications that improve sleep latency include zolpidem, eszopiclone, zaleplon, and zopiclone (not available in the United States). Additionally, eszopiclone improves maintenance of sleep.[68,69] Their effects on various aspects of performance vary depending on the duration of sleep and medication half-life.

Immediate effects after ingestion, without sleep, include impairments in memory, attention, and psychomotor tasks.[70,71] These measures may also be affected by restricted sleep duration (eg, interrupted sleep), and tend to be more pronounced with long-acting zopiclone (half-life 6 hours), more moderate with zolpidem (half-life 2.5 hours), and minimal with zalpelon (half-life 1 hour).[72–76] Minimal to zero impairments on either the aforementioned tasks or on measures of performance have been noted for zolpidem or zalpelon after a full 8-hour sleep period.[77–79] Eszopiclone is a relatively newer agent and data are sparse; however, given its relatively longer half-life (6 hours), it may be reasonable to anticipate effects on performance analogous to zopiclone administration.

Pragmatic considerations are recommended before the use of these or any other agents to minimize effects on athletic performance. Restricted use preceding competition (especially in athletes unaccustomed to hypnotic use), a comprehensive awareness of potential side effects, and selected restriction to these medications (ie, ensuring the possibility of a full sleep period before use) are all important factors.[80] And although their abuse potential is notably limited compared with benzodiazepines, these medications may also be used "recreationally," which further underscores the need for close monitoring.

Concerns regarding the increased risk for various medical problems with nonbenzodiazepine use have been addressed. Of greatest pertinence to athletes are worsening gastroesophageal reflux, decrements in immune system performance, and increased risk of cancer. Elite athletes, particularly those engaging in endurance events, are commonly affected by gastroesophageal reflux disease (GERD) secondary to altered gastrointestinal function and mechanical effects.[81] Moreover, Gagliardi and colleagues[82] have shown that zolpidem reduces the protective arousal response to nocturnal acid, significantly increases nocturnal exposure time to acid, and increases the duration of individual acid reflux events in both healthy individuals and those with

GERD. Thus, athletes with underlying GERD who use zolpidem may have an increased risk for complicated disease.

Endurance athletes may also have immune system dysfunction.[83] Although not clinically immunocompromised, extended strenuous training may result in decrements in immune system performance, thus rendering these athletes more prone to minor disease processes, such as upper respiratory infections. A recent meta-analysis by Joya and colleagues[84] demonstrated a risk ratio of 1.44 for developing an infection following the administration of a nonbenzodiazepine medication compared with a placebo group. This finding is of particular importance, both within the context of the findings of Gagliardi and colleagues[82] and the association of GERD and upper respiratory tract infections.

Finally, the nonbenzodiazepine sleep aids have been associated with an increased risk of cancer, particularly skin cancer, such as basal cell carcinoma.[85] Although an underlying mechanism has not been proposed, these are relatively important implications for endurance athletes given their generally higher than average amount of sun exposure and relative immune system dysfunction. It should be noted that these are preliminary and perhaps negligible associations, especially when these agents are used only occasionally (eg, in the setting of transmeridian travel). Affirmative studies are needed; however, it is important for the medical staff to be aware of these possible adverse effects.

Stimulants

Stimulants, including caffeine, modafinil, and dextroamphetamine, have garnered interest as a means to combat cognitive decrements related to sleep deprivation and JL. Caffeine, in both regular and sustained-release formulas at doses below the threshold necessary to inhibit fine-motor performance, has been shown to be effective at improving measures of attention and reaction time with shift work and transmeridian travel.[86,87] Caffeine is also known to provide a tangible benefit to endurance and high-intensity exercise performance under "normal" conditions,[88] and may possess chronobiotic properties that facilitate re-entrainment.[89] Similar to melatonin, OTC supplements and high-energy drinks should be used with great caution by the high-performance athlete to prevent unintentional ingestion of restricted substances. The effects of stimulants, such as modafinil and dextroamphetamine, have been examined in other populations of interest, but use of these medications is obviously limited in athletes because of restrictions imposed by WADA and USADA (as discussed elsewhere in this article).

Considerations in Special Populations and Circumstances

The youth athlete

Following travel, the young athlete may have relatively better tolerance to the uncomfortable side effects of JL,[90] yet may have specific difficulty with phase re-entrainment and adjusting to a new sleep cycle.[91] Although research in this area is inadequate, slower shifts in sleep habits and diurnal performance should be considered by the medical staff when planning transmeridian travel. Adolescents are also more prone to have baseline circadian rhythms that are relatively "shifted" toward the evening,[92] which could affect the timing of re-entrainment strategies. Pharmacologic agents should be used with extreme caution. Melatonin has not been evaluated in controlled studies for treating JL in children, and may have physiologic implications beyond those observed in adults.[91] Although somewhat controversial, there have been reports that melatonin may lower the seizure threshold, and its use should be closely monitored in youth populations.[63]

The masters athlete
The physiology of the circadian rhythm changes with aging, with reduced levels of exogenous melatonin production and deterioration of the suprachiasmatic nuclei.[93] As a result, older individuals tend to have a weaker level of synchronization of rhythms because of impaired responsiveness of the "central clock" to external cues.[94] Thus, the masters athlete may be particularly sensitive to the effects of JL,[2] and may also have altered responses to some of the management strategies discussed. For example, older individuals appear to have a reduced dose-response to a range of intense light[95] with blunted improvements in alertness, sleepiness, and mood.[96] In contrast to the youth athlete, the circadian rhythms of older individuals tend to become phase advanced, and this fact also should be taken into account when planning management strategies.

Pharmacologic agents should also be used with increased caution. This age group has been shown to be responsive to the positive effects of melatonin on sleep characteristics and producing phase shifts; however, melatonin may cause reductions in blood pressure, increase intraocular pressure, and increase clotting activity,[63] all of which may have implications in the masters athlete with transmeridian travel. Furthermore, the use of sleep aids has been noted to be correlated with fall and fracture risk[70,97] and may potentiate cognitive side effects when used with other medications such as melatonin.[73]

The female athlete
Gender differences with respect to sleep have been noted, with females demonstrating an earlier onset of increase in endogenous melatonin relative to sleep.[98] This observation dictates the importance of making adjustments to the timing of melatonin administration in female athletes. Melatonin may also have various endocrine effects, and should be avoided in those who are either pregnant or are attempting to become pregnant.[63] The safety of exogenous melatonin during breast-feeding has not been established.

Ethnic differences
Ethnic differences in circadian rhythm have recently been noted. Compared with Caucasians, individuals of African descent possess a circadian clock with a shorter periodicity.[99] This difference translates to a relatively lower ability of Caucasians to undergo phase advances and a higher relative ability to undergo phase delays.[99] This phenomenon is independent of iris color.[100] These differences may be considerations when planning travel re-entrainment strategies during both eastward and westward travel.

Future Directions

As previously discussed, the vast majority of current knowledge regarding the problem of JL and its management is reliant on a relatively small collection of studies, few of which were performed in a "real-world" clinical setting of JL. Additional studies in athletic and other populations in "real" and controlled environments are necessary to strengthen the existing evidence regarding the effects of JL on athletic performance, its effects on health and wellness, and the efficacy of current management strategies. These studies may also be extended to determine how manipulation of circadian rhythms can be used to time low or high core temperatures for improved performance and reduced health risks in varied climates.[11]

New interventions and strategies to minimize and reverse symptoms of JL expeditiously should be considered. For example, nutrition is a pivotal factor in peak athletic performance, but little knowledge exists regarding the effects of different nutritional strategies on JL symptoms and re-entrainment,[101] even though gastrointestinal distress, reduced appetite, and altered dietary habits are common presenting features of JL. New pharmacologic options are being developed, including the melatonin receptor agonist agomelatine, and various serotonin receptor antagonists,[102–104] which may also play a role in altering sleep characteristics. Improved basic science knowledge of the interaction and physiologic relationship of central and peripheral circadian clocks may also lead to additional, novel therapies for JL to improve sleep and quicken re-entrainment.[105]

UPDATES ON ANTI-DOPING POLICIES

WADA and USADA are dynamic organizations that endorse, direct, and supervise the constantly evolving crusade against doping in all sports. The recommended regulations and restrictions, in response to the best available medical evidence and monitored "substance use" patterns across sports, changes periodically. Several alterations to "permitted" use of medications and the necessary documentation to support the use of medications have been made by WADA and USADA in recent years. It is therefore imperative for athletes, staff, and medical teams to maintain and update their base knowledge on subtle changes in WADA and USADA policies to preserve legal, competitive status.

The focus of this section is to briefly outline and discuss the recent, important advances on the rationale of WADA and USADA for selected medical interventions, drugs, and monitoring. Updates on specific topics include the appropriate and timely submission of Therapeutic Use Exemption (TUE) forms by physicians, use of stimulants (including pseudoephedrine), medications used for exercise-induced bronchoconstriction, alcohol, beta-blockers, changes in the status of platelet-rich plasma therapy, and alterations to the "Athlete Whereabouts" system for out-of-competition testing. It is beyond the scope of this article to discuss the vast lists of prohibited substances and numerous nuances associated with medication use in competitive athletes; however, physicians caring for international athletes should be familiar with WADA's updated 2011 prohibited list of medications and are encouraged to carry an updated 2011 "wallet card" (published by USADA) that has a detailed list of "prohibited" and "not prohibited" substances and methods for athletes both "in and out of competition." For a complete review and to download these important resources, please refer to the following comprehensive, informative Web sites[106,107]:

1. WADA: www.wada-ama.org
2. USADA: www.usantidoping.org.

Therapeutic Use Exemption

A Therapeutic Use Exemption (TUE) grants athletes "special permission" to use a prohibited substance for medical reasons based on substantial and specific medical documentation. A TUE is typically required for all prohibited substances and methods as outlined by WADA and USADA. However, requirements for timely submission of TUEs vary depending on the athlete's competition status. For example, athletes competing at international events (sanctioned by the international federation of their specific sport) who are part of the USADA or International Federation Testing Pool must submit a TUE in advance of using any prohibited substance, regardless of competition level. Failure to do so may result in an anti-doping violation.

TUEs can be obtained from the USADA Web site. Two documents should be downloaded and completed. First, an application form should be filled out by the athlete and reviewed by the physician. Second, the physician should fill out a medical information form that justifies the medical use of the prohibited substance. Both forms should be returned to USADA by facsimile or electronic mail.

Medications

Stimulants

All stimulants are prohibited with the exception of imidazole derivatives for topical use, and those listed on the 2011 Monitoring Program, including bupropion, caffeine, phenylephrine, phenylpropanolamine, pipradrol, pseudoephedrine (prohibited for "in-competition" use at urinary concentrations above 150 µg/mL), and synephrine. TUEs are needed for all athletes diagnosed and treated with stimulants for either attention deficit disorder or attention deficit hyperactivity disorder. Athletes with narcolepsy who have been prescribed modafinil or armodafinil also need a TUE. Finally, a nutritional supplement commonly referred to as "geranium oil" or "geranium root extract" contains a stimulant "methylhexaneamine. " This substance is currently included on WADA's Prohibited List as a *specified* substance.

Pseudoephedrine

Pseudoephedrine is a stimulant found in numerous OTC medications and is commonly used as a decongestant to treat symptoms of upper respiratory illnesses and environmental allergies. It was previously on the prohibited list until 2003, when it was removed from the list based on an acknowledged lack of evidence of its ergogenic effects at therapeutic doses.[108–112] Subsequently, it was added to WADA's Monitoring Program. Since 2003, a significant increase in its use in several sports and various levels of competition has been noted.[113–115] Furthermore, additional knowledge regarding the performance-enhancing effects of pseudoephedrine at supratherapeutic doses has been revealing. Pseudoephedrine has been shown to acutely increase simple measures of strength, power, and lung function,[116] and improve both running and cycling time trials.[111,117] Secondary to its "pattern of use" and growing evidence for ergogenic effects at high doses, it was reintroduced in 2010 as a prohibited stimulant for "in-competition" use at urinary concentrations higher than 150 µg/mL. Thus, based on individual differences in metabolism and clearance rates, pseudoephedrine use should be discontinued 24 hours before the "time of day" considered by sporting organizations as "in-competition" time.

Additionally, sports medicine staff should educate athletes about 2 critical facts. First, pseudoephedrine is an ingredient in several OTC preparations and, second, that 24 hours may not be enough time for pseudoephedrine to be excreted from the body. Thus, it is imperative that athletes refrain from the use of all medications during "in-competition." And if medications are absolutely necessary, medical staff should evaluate the ingredients of all medications before use by athletes.

Medications for exercise-induced bronchoconstriction

Beta 2 agonists can induce bronchial smooth muscle relaxation, exert anabolic effects, and produce arterial dilation in skeletal muscles, enhance glycogenolysis and gluconeogenesis, and inhibit release of chemical mediators of inflammation from mast cells. Accordingly, *all* oral beta 2 agonists are prohibited. Inhaled beta 2 agonists are also prohibited and require a TUE *except for* salbutamol (albuterol in the United States; dosage under 1600 µg in 24 hours) and salmeterol. Notably, athletes who in addition to albuterol also need to use and have a TUE for medications that are categorized as either "diuretics" or "masking agents," need a TUE for albuterol. Additionally, effective January 1, 2011, athletes do not have to declare inhaled asthma medications (albuterol, salmeterol, inhaled glucocorticoids, such as fluticasone and budesonide) to USADA or their international federations. However, athletes still need to list these medications on the Declaration of Record (DCOR) form at the time of anti-doping testing.

Athletes should also be counseled on the critical need to examine their inhaler closely to determine the dosage delivered with each puff, because the threshold (1600 µg in 24 hours) may translate into a large range of doses. Also, some inhalers have more than one active ingredient, one of which may need a TUE application. Thus, before use, it is advisable to have athletes consult www.GlobalDRO.com to assess if their inhalers contain medications that need a TUE.

Alcohol

In 2011, WADA has removed alcohol from their list of prohibited substances for Modern Pentathlon (for disciplines involving shooting). This change was based on a request by the Union Internationale de Pentathlon Moderne (UIPM) secondary to changes in the format of the competition.

Beta-blockers

In 2011, in response to requests by 2 sports federations, WADA has added beta-blockers to their list of prohibited substances for Skeleton (governed by Fédération Internationale de Bobsleigh et de Tobogganing [FIBT]) and Darts (governed by the World Darts Federation [WDF]). However, following a recent request by the Fédération Internationale de Gymnastique (FIG) to WADA, beta-blockers are no longer prohibited in gymnastics.

Platelet-Rich Plasma

Platelet-Rich Plasma (PRP) is a treatment used for a variety of musculoskeletal conditions, which consists of the local delivery of a concentrated, autologous platelet preparation. This technique has been rapidly gaining attention and popularity in the field of sports medicine as a means to potentiate and hasten recovery from athletic injury. The underlying physiologic basis of PRP is to deliver a localized burst of growth factors to injured tissue. Platelets contain a variety of growth factors that are released at the site of injury, including unbound insulinlike growth factor-1 (IGF-1), platelet-derived growth factor, vascular-endothelial growth factor, basic fibroblast growth factor, epidermal growth factor, and transforming growth factor beta 1.[118] Furthermore, the plasma component of the PRP preparation contains hepatocyte growth factor and IGF-1, the vast majority of which is protein-bound.

The primary focus from a doping perspective has been IGF-1, which exerts its systemic anabolic effects by stimulating skeletal muscle hypertrophy and increasing availability of glucose to skeletal muscle.[119] As a result, the use of PRP via intramuscular injection was listed as a prohibited substance by WADA, and the use of PRP for the injection in other tissues formerly required a TUE.

However, some characteristics of PRP have cast doubt on its potential use for performance enhancement.[120] The unbound, active form of IGF-1 has a very short half-life (10 minutes), which is unlikely to be long enough to allow for any systemic effects. Additionally, the dose of IGF-1 used for producing systemic effects is 2 orders of magnitude greater than that delivered via PRP. Furthermore, preliminary evidence has also demonstrated a lack of clinically significant, systemic impact on levels of a limited set of growth factors after PRP injections.[121] Based on the available evidence, WADA has removed PRP injections from the Prohibited List for 2011.

Athlete Whereabouts

"Athlete Whereabouts" is the WADA system used to track athletes to effectively test them "out-of-competition." In 2006, WADA engaged in a 3-year review of the system, partially for the purpose of standardizing the provision of rules and consequences of missed tests. The new rules for the Athlete Whereabouts system were subsequently introduced in 2009.

Previously, athletes were required to specify their location for testing 90 days in advance. They were required to be available for 1 hour a day, 5 days a week, and were required to be present at the indicated location for only a "portion" of the specified hour. Comparatively, the new rules that took effect in 2009 required athletes to be available for testing 7 days a week, for the "full" hour. Expectedly, these changes were controversial, as athletes and governing bodies of various sports provoked ethical and legal concerns regarding the limits of the athletes' right to privacy. WADA is currently engaged in a 1-year review to assess the impact of these changes, and have cited significant, broad support through stakeholder surveys. The medical staff and athletes should remain vigilant for any potential changes to the program as WADA proceeds with and completes the review.

SUMMARY

The current knowledge regarding the effects of JL on athletic performance and its management is not robust. Additional insights may be reasonably inferred from studies in nonathletes and those individuals with altered "schedule shifts" or sleep disorders. The negative effects of JL may be best reduced by adopting a multimodality approach using pretravel schedule shifting, appropriately timed *zeitgebers*, and the judicious use of melatonin and other pharmacologic agents to aid re-entrainment and improve sleep characteristics. Attention may also be directed to the timing of exercise to further aid re-entrainment, and align training and diurnal rhythms of performance to competition schedule in the new "time zone." An appreciation of the basic chronobiology of JL is critical to the efficacy of these interventions. The foundation of any management strategy must be rooted in thoughtful, advanced planning by the medical team and appropriate education of the athletes and support staff.

Based on evolving science and patterns of medication use, both WADA and USADA have recently made specific changes regarding the use of stimulants (including pseudoephedrine), information regarding the use of medications for exercise-induced bronchoconstriction, alcohol and beta-blockers, and PRP. Based on ethical and legal concerns, pragmatics of the Athlete Whereabouts system are being reviewed to improve monitoring protocols fairly while ensuring compliance. Because of intermittent changes in WADA and USADA rules, it is critical that medical staff maintain familiarity and awareness on a continual basis to effectively educate athletes and support staff. Detailed information on policies and procedures can be obtained at WADA's Web site, www.wada-ama.org, and at USADA's Web site at www.usantidoping.org.

REFERENCES

1. Aschoff J, Hoffmann K, Pohl H, et al. Re-entrainment of circadian rhythms after phase-shifts of the Zeitgeber. Chronobiologia 1975;2(1):23–78.
2. Monk TH. Aging human circadian rhythms: conventional wisdom may not always be right. J Biol Rhythms 2005;20(4):366–74.
3. Monk TH, Buysse DJ, Carrier J, et al. Inducing jet-lag in older people: directional asymmetry. J Sleep Res 2000;9(2):101–16.

4. Reilly T, Waterhouse J, Edwards B. Jet lag and air travel: implications for performance. Clin Sports Med 2005;24(2):367–80, xii.
5. Waterhouse J, Reilly T, Atkinson G, et al. Jet lag: trends and coping strategies. Lancet 2007;369(9567):1117–29.
6. Kovac J, Husse J, Oster H. A time to fast, a time to feast: the crosstalk between metabolism and the circadian clock. Mol Cells 2009;28(2):75–80.
7. Vansteensel MJ, Michel S, Meijer JH. Organization of cell and tissue circadian pacemakers: a comparison among species. Brain Res Rev 2008;58(1):18–47.
8. Dibner C, Schibler U, Albrecht U. The mammalian circadian timing system: organization and coordination of central and peripheral clocks. Annu Rev Physiol 2010;72:517–49.
9. Revell VL, Eastman CI. How to trick mother nature into letting you fly around or stay up all night. J Biol Rhythms 2005;20(4):353–65.
10. Murray G, Nicholas CL, Kleiman J, et al. Nature's clocks and human mood: the circadian system modulates reward motivation. Emotion 2009;9(5):705–16.
11. Reilly T, Atkinson G, Gregson W, et al. Some chronobiological considerations related to physical exercise. Clin Ter 2006;157(3):249–64.
12. Kline CE, Durstine JL, Davis JM, et al. Circadian variation in swim performance. J Appl Physiol 2007;102(2):641–9.
13. Reilly T, Edwards B. Altered sleep-wake cycles and physical performance in athletes. Physiol Behav 2007;90(2–3):274–84.
14. Drust B, Waterhouse J, Atkinson G, et al. Circadian rhythms in sports performance—an update. Chronobiol Int 2005;22(1):21–44.
15. Bullock N, Martin DT, Ross A, et al. Effect of long haul travel on maximal sprint performance and diurnal variations in elite skeleton athletes. Br J Sports Med 2007;41(9):569–73 [discussion: 573].
16. Bambaeichi E, Reilly T, Cable NT, et al. Influence of time of day and partial sleep loss on muscle strength in eumenorrheic females. Ergonomics 2005;48(11–14): 1499–511.
17. Akerstedt T. Altered sleep/wake patterns and mental performance. Physiol Behav 2007;90(2/3):209–18.
18. Thacker SB, Gilchrist J, Stroup DF, et al. The impact of stretching on sports injury risk: a systematic review of the literature. Med Sci Sports Exerc 2004; 36(3):371–8.
19. Witvrouw E, Mahieu N, Danneels L, et al. Stretching and injury prevention: an obscure relationship. Sports Med 2004;34(7):443–9.
20. Swanik CB, Covassin T, Stearne DJ, et al. The relationship between neurocognitive function and noncontact anterior cruciate ligament injuries. Am J Sports Med 2007;35(6):943–8.
21. Taimela S, Osterman L, Kujala U, et al. Motor ability and personality with reference to soccer injuries. J Sports Med Phys Fitness 1990;30(2):194–201.
22. Taimela S. Relation between speed of reaction and psychometric tests of mental ability in musculoskeletal injury-prone subjects. Percept Mot Skills 1990;70(1): 155–61.
23. Atkinson G, Drust B, George K, et al. Chronobiological considerations for exercise and heart disease. Sports Med 2006;36(6):487–500.
24. Elliot DL, Goldberg L, Kuehl KS. Young women's anterior cruciate ligament injuries: an expanded model and prevention paradigm. Sports Med 2010; 40(5):367–76.
25. Eastman CI, Gazda CJ, Burgess HJ, et al. Advancing circadian rhythms before eastward flight: a strategy to prevent or reduce jet lag. Sleep 2005;28(1):33–44.

26. Eastman CI, Burgess HJ. How to travel the world without jet lag. Sleep Med Clin 2009;4(2):241–55.
27. Revell VL, Burgess HJ, Gazda CJ, et al. Advancing human circadian rhythms with afternoon melatonin and morning intermittent bright light. J Clin Endocrinol Metab 2006;91(1):54–9.
28. Burgess HJ, Crowley SJ, Gazda CJ, et al. Preflight adjustment to eastward travel: 3 days of advancing sleep with and without morning bright light. J Biol Rhythms 2003;18(4):318–28.
29. Ficca G, Axelsson J, Mollicone DJ, et al. Naps, cognition and performance. Sleep Med Rev 2010;14(4):249–58.
30. Waterhouse J, Atkinson G, Edwards B, et al. The role of a short post-lunch nap in improving cognitive, motor, and sprint performance in participants with partial sleep deprivation. J Sports Sci 2007;25(14):1557–66.
31. Atkinson G, Edwards B, Reilly T, et al. Exercise as a synchroniser of human circadian rhythms: an update and discussion of the methodological problems. Eur J Appl Physiol 2007;99(4):331–41.
32. Montaruli A, Roveda E, Calogiuri G, et al. The sportsman readjustment after transcontinental flight: a study on marathon runners. J Sports Med Phys Fitness 2009;49(4):372–81.
33. Yamanaka Y, Hashimoto S, Tanahashi Y, et al. Physical exercise accelerates re-entrainment of human sleep-wake cycle but not of plasma melatonin rhythm to 8-h phase-advanced sleep schedule. Am J Physiol Regul Integr Comp Physiol 2010;298(3):R681–91.
34. Smith MR, Fogg LF, Eastman CI. Practical interventions to promote circadian adaptation to permanent night shift work: study 4. J Biol Rhythms 2009;24(2):161–72.
35. Santhi N, Aeschbach D, Horowitz TS, et al. The impact of sleep timing and bright light exposure on attentional impairment during night work. J Biol Rhythms 2008;23(4):341–52.
36. Paul MA, Miller JC, Love RJ, et al. Timing light treatment for eastward and westward travel preparation. Chronobiol Int 2009;26(5):867–90.
37. Cardinali DP, Bortman GP, Liotta G, et al. A multifactorial approach employing melatonin to accelerate resynchronization of sleep-wake cycle after a 12 time-zone westerly transmeridian flight in elite soccer athletes. J Pineal Res 2002; 32(1):41–6.
38. Cardinali DP, Furio AM, Reyes MP, et al. The use of chronobiotics in the resynchronization of the sleep-wake cycle. Cancer Causes Control 2006;17(4):601–9.
39. Crowley SJ, Lee C, Tseng CY, et al. Combinations of bright light, scheduled dark, sunglasses, and melatonin to facilitate circadian entrainment to night shift work. J Biol Rhythms 2003;18(6):513–23.
40. Boulos Z, Macchi MM, Stürchler MP, et al. Light visor treatment for jet lag after westward travel across six time zones. Aviat Space Environ Med 2002;73(10): 953–63.
41. Yoon IY, Jeong DU, Kwon KB, et al. Bright light exposure at night and light attenuation in the morning improve adaptation of night shift workers. Sleep 2002; 25(3):351–6.
42. Kripke DF, Elliott JA, Youngstedt SD, et al. Circadian phase response curves to light in older and young women and men. J Circadian Rhythms 2007;5:4.
43. Phipps-Nelson J, Redman JR, Schlangen LJ, et al. Blue light exposure reduces objective measures of sleepiness during prolonged nighttime performance testing. Chronobiol Int 2009;26(5):891–912.

44. Revell VL, Arendt J, Fogg LF, et al. Alerting effects of light are sensitive to very short wavelengths. Neurosci Lett 2006;399(1/2):96–100.
45. Gooley JJ, Rajaratnam SM, Brainard GC, et al. Spectral responses of the human circadian system depend on the irradiance and duration of exposure to light. Sci Transl Med 2010;2(31):31ra33.
46. Revell VL, Barrett DC, Schlangen LJ, et al. Predicting human nocturnal nonvisual responses to monochromatic and polychromatic light with a melanopsin photosensitivity function. Chronobiol Int 2010;27(9/10):1762–77.
47. Wright HR, Lack LC. Effect of light wavelength on suppression and phase delay of the melatonin rhythm. Chronobiol Int 2001;18(5):801–8.
48. Smith MR, Eastman CI. Phase delaying the human circadian clock with blue-enriched polychromatic light. Chronobiol Int 2009;26(4):709–25.
49. Smith MR, Revell VL, Eastman CI. Phase advancing the human circadian clock with blue-enriched polychromatic light. Sleep Med 2009;10(3):287–94.
50. Sack RL, Auckley D, Auger RR, et al. Circadian rhythm sleep disorders: part I, basic principles, shift work and jet lag disorders. An American Academy of Sleep Medicine review. Sleep 2007;30(11):1460–83.
51. Richardson GS, Zee PC, Wang-Weigand S, et al. Circadian phase-shifting effects of repeated ramelteon administration in healthy adults. J Clin Sleep Med 2008;4(5):456–61.
52. Paul MA, Miller JC, Gray GW, et al. Melatonin treatment for eastward and westward travel preparation. Psychopharmacology (Berl) 2010;208(3):377–86.
53. Paul MA, Gray GW, Lieberman HR, et al. Phase advance with separate and combined melatonin and light treatment. Psychopharmacology (Berl) 2010;214(2):515–23.
54. Atkinson G, Drust B, Reilly T, et al. The relevance of melatonin to sports medicine and science. Sports Med 2003;33(11):809–31.
55. Atkinson G, Holder A, Robertson C, et al. Effects of daytime ingestion of melatonin on short-term athletic performance. Ergonomics 2005;48(11–14):1512–22.
56. Graw P, Werth E, Kräuchi K, et al. Early morning melatonin administration impairs psychomotor vigilance. Behav Brain Res 2001;121(1/2):167–72.
57. Mero AA, Vähälummukka M, Hulmi JJ, et al. Effects of resistance exercise session after oral ingestion of melatonin on physiological and performance responses of adult men. Eur J Appl Physiol 2006;96(6):729–39.
58. Storm WF, Eddy DR, Welch CB, et al. Cognitive performance following premature awakening from zolpidem or melatonin induced daytime sleep. Aviat Space Environ Med 2007;78(1):10–20.
59. Wesensten NJ, Balkin TJ, Reichardt RM, et al. Daytime sleep and performance following a zolpidem and melatonin cocktail. Sleep 2005;28(1):93–103.
60. Paul MA, Gray G, Kenny G, et al. Impact of melatonin, zaleplon, zopiclone, and temazepam on psychomotor performance. Aviat Space Environ Med 2003;74(12):1263–70.
61. Kitajima T, Kanbayashi T, Saitoh Y, et al. The effects of oral melatonin on the autonomic function in healthy subjects. Psychiatry Clin Neurosci 2001;55(3):299–300.
62. Nishiyama K, Yasue H, Moriyama Y, et al. Acute effects of melatonin administration on cardiovascular autonomic regulation in healthy men. Am Heart J 2001;141(5):E9.
63. Melatonin: professional monograph. Natural Standard. 2010. Available at: http://naturalstandard.com/databases/herbssupplements/melatonin.asp#. Accessed November 1, 2010.

64. Kato K, Hirai K, Nishiyama K, et al. Neurochemical properties of ramelteon (TAK-375), a selective MT1/MT2 receptor agonist. Neuropharmacology 2005;48(2):301–10.
65. Rajaratnam SM, Polymeropoulos MH, Fisher DM, et al. Melatonin agonist tasimelteon (VEC-162) for transient insomnia after sleep-time shift: two randomised controlled multicentre trials. Lancet 2009;373(9662):482–91.
66. Zee PC, Wang-Weigand S, Wright KP, et al. Effects of ramelteon on insomnia symptoms induced by rapid, eastward travel. Sleep Med 2010;11(6):525–33.
67. Burgess HJ, Eastman CI. Short nights reduce light-induced circadian phase delays in humans. Sleep 2006;29(1):25–30.
68. Dundar Y, Dodd S, Stroble J, et al. Comparative efficacy of newer hypnotic drugs for the short-term management of insomnia: a systematic review and meta-analysis. Hum Psychopharmacol 2004;19(5):305–22.
69. Morin AK, Willett K. The role of eszopiclone in the treatment of insomnia. Adv Ther 2009;26(5):500–18.
70. Terzano MG, Rossi M, Palomba V, et al. New drugs for insomnia: comparative tolerability of zopiclone, zolpidem and zaleplon. Drug Saf 2003;26(4):261–82.
71. Vermeeren A. Residual effects of hypnotics: epidemiology and clinical implications. CNS Drugs 2004;18(5):297–328.
72. Leufkens TR, Lund JS, Vermeeren A. Highway driving performance and cognitive functioning the morning after bedtime and middle-of-the-night use of gaboxadol, zopiclone and zolpidem. J Sleep Res 2009;18(4):387–96.
73. Otmani S, Demazières A, Staner C, et al. Effects of prolonged-release melatonin, zolpidem, and their combination on psychomotor functions, memory recall, and driving skills in healthy middle aged and elderly volunteers. Hum Psychopharmacol 2008;23(8):693–705.
74. Hindmarch I, Patat A, Stanley N, et al. Residual effects of zaleplon and zolpidem following middle of the night administration five hours to one hour before awakening. Hum Psychopharmacol 2001;16(2):159–67.
75. Verster JC, Volkerts ER, Schreuder AH, et al. Residual effects of middle-of-the-night administration of zaleplon and zolpidem on driving ability, memory functions, and psychomotor performance. J Clin Psychopharmacol 2002;22(6):576–83.
76. Danjou P, Paty I, Fruncillo R, et al. A comparison of the residual effects of zaleplon and zolpidem following administration 5 to 2 h before awakening. Br J Clin Pharmacol 1999;48(3):367–74.
77. Blin O, Micallef J, Audebert C, et al. A double-blind, placebo- and flurazepam-controlled investigation of the residual psychomotor and cognitive effects of modified release zolpidem in young healthy volunteers. J Clin Psychopharmacol 2006;26(3):284–9.
78. Hindmarch I, Legangneux E, Stanley N, et al. A double-blind, placebo-controlled investigation of the residual psychomotor and cognitive effects of zolpidem-MR in healthy elderly volunteers. Br J Clin Pharmacol 2006;62(5):538–45.
79. Roth T, Soubrane C, Titeux L, et al. Efficacy and safety of zolpidem-MR: a double-blind, placebo-controlled study in adults with primary insomnia. Sleep Med 2006;7(5):397–406.
80. Verster JC, Volkerts ER, Olivier B, et al. Zolpidem and traffic safety—the importance of treatment compliance. Curr Drug Saf 2007;2(3):220–6.
81. Parmelee-Peters K, Moeller JL. Gastroesophageal reflux in athletes. Curr Sports Med Rep 2004;3(2):107–11.

82. Gagliardi GS, Shah AP, Goldstein M, et al. Effect of zolpidem on the sleep arousal response to nocturnal esophageal acid exposure. Clin Gastroenterol Hepatol 2009;7(9):948–52.

83. Brolinson PG, Elliott D. Exercise and the immune system. Clin Sports Med 2007; 26(3):311–9.

84. Joya FL, Kripke DF, Loving RT, et al. Meta-analyses of hypnotics and infections: eszopiclone, ramelteon, zaleplon, and zolpidem. J Clin Sleep Med 2009;5(4): 377–83.

85. Kripke DF. Possibility that certain hypnotics might cause cancer in skin. J Sleep Res 2008;17(3):245–50.

86. Beaumont M, Batéjat D, Piérard C, et al. Caffeine or melatonin effects on sleep and sleepiness after rapid eastward transmeridian travel. J Appl Physiol 2004; 96(1):50–8.

87. Schweitzer PK, Randazzo AC, Stone K, et al. Laboratory and field studies of naps and caffeine as practical countermeasures for sleep-wake problems associated with night work. Sleep 2006;29(1):39–50.

88. Goldstein ER, Ziegenfuss T, Kalman D, et al. International society of sports nutrition position stand: caffeine and performance. J Int Soc Sports Nutr 2010;7(1):5.

89. Pierard C, Beaumont M, Enslen M, et al. Resynchronization of hormonal rhythms after an eastbound flight in humans: effects of slow-release caffeine and melatonin. Eur J Appl Physiol 2001;85(1/2):144–50.

90. Moline ML, Pollak CP, Monk TH, et al. Age-related differences in recovery from simulated jet lag. Sleep 1992;15(1):28–40.

91. Stauffer WM, Konop RJ, Kamat D. Traveling with infants and young children. Part I: anticipatory guidance: travel preparation and preventive health advice. J Travel Med 2001;8(5):254–9.

92. Roenneberg T, Kuehnle T, Pramstaller PP, et al. A marker for the end of adolescence. Curr Biol 2004;14(24):R1038–9.

93. Touitou Y. Human aging and melatonin. Clinical relevance. Exp Gerontol 2001; 36(7):1083–100.

94. Swaab DF, Fliers E, Partiman TS. The suprachiasmatic nucleus of the human brain in relation to sex, age and senile dementia. Brain Res 1985;342(1):37–44.

95. Duffy JF, Zeitzer JM, Czeisler CA. Decreased sensitivity to phase-delaying effects of moderate intensity light in older subjects. Neurobiol Aging 2007; 28(5):799–807.

96. Sletten TL, Revell VL, Middleton B, et al. Age-related changes in acute and phase-advancing responses to monochromatic light. J Biol Rhythms 2009; 24(1):73–84.

97. Allain H, Bentué-Ferrer D, Polard E, et al. Postural instability and consequent falls and hip fractures associated with use of hypnotics in the elderly: a comparative review. Drugs Aging 2005;22(9):749–65.

98. Cain SW, Dennison CF, Zeitzer JM, et al. Sex differences in phase angle of entrainment and melatonin amplitude in humans. J Biol Rhythms 2010;25(4): 288–96.

99. Smith MR, Burgess HJ, Fogg LF, et al. Racial differences in the human endogenous circadian period. PLoS One 2009;4(6):e6014.

100. Canton JL, Smith MR, Choi HS, et al. Phase delaying the human circadian clock with a single light pulse and moderate delay of the sleep/dark episode: no influence of iris color. J Circadian Rhythms 2009;7:8.

101. Armstrong LE. Nutritional strategies for football: counteracting heat, cold, high altitude, and jet lag. J Sports Sci 2006;24(7):723–40.

102. Srinivasan V, Singh J, Pandi-Perumal SR, et al. Jet lag, circadian rhythm sleep disturbances, and depression: the role of melatonin and its analogs. Adv Ther 2010;27(11):796–813.
103. Yannielli P, Harrington ME. Let there be "more" light: enhancement of light actions on the circadian system through non-photic pathways. Prog Neurobiol 2004;74(1):59–76.
104. Sterniczuk R, Stepkowski A, Jones M, et al. Enhancement of photic shifts with the 5-HT1A mixed agonist/antagonist NAN-190: intra-suprachiasmatic nucleus pathway. Neuroscience 2008;153(3):571–80.
105. Kiessling S, Eichele G, Oster H. Adrenal glucocorticoids have a key role in circadian resynchronization in a mouse model of jet lag. J Clin Invest 2010;120(7): 2600–9.
106. Available at: www.usantidoping.org. Accessed January 15, 2011.
107. Available at: www.wada-ama.org. Accessed January 15, 2011.
108. Gillies H, Derman WE, Noakes TD, et al. Pseudoephedrine is without ergogenic effects during prolonged exercise. J Appl Physiol 1996;81(6):2611–7.
109. Clemons JM, Crosby SL. Cardiopulmonary and subjective effects of a 60 mg dose of pseudoephedrine on graded treadmill exercise. J Sports Med Phys Fitness 1993;33(4):405–12.
110. Swain RA, Harsha DM, Baenziger J, et al. Do pseudoephedrine or phenylpropanolamine improve maximum oxygen uptake and time to exhaustion? Clin J Sport Med 1997;7(3):168–73.
111. Hodges AN, Lynn BM, Bula JE, et al. Effects of pseudoephedrine on maximal cycling power and submaximal cycling efficiency. Med Sci Sports Exerc 2003;35(8):1316–9.
112. Chester N, Reilly T, Mottram DR. Physiological, subjective and performance effects of pseudoephedrine and phenylpropanolamine during endurance running exercise. Int J Sports Med 2003;24(1):3–8.
113. Bents RT, Tokish JM, Goldberg L. Ephedrine, pseudoephedrine, and amphetamine prevalence in college hockey players: most report performance-enhancing use. Phys Sportsmed 2004;32(9):30–4.
114. Bents RT, Marsh E. Patterns of ephedra and other stimulant use in collegiate hockey athletes. Int J Sport Nutr Exerc Metab 2006;16(6):636–43.
115. Pokrywka A, Tszyrsznic W, Kwiatkowska DJ. Problems of the use of pseudoephedrine by athletes. Int J Sports Med 2009;30(8):569–72.
116. Gill ND, Shield A, Blazevich AJ, et al. Muscular and cardiorespiratory effects of pseudoephedrine in human athletes. Br J Clin Pharmacol 2000;50(3):205–13.
117. Pritchard-Peschek KR, Jenkins DG, Osborne MA, et al. Pseudoephedrine ingestion and cycling time-trial performance. Int J Sport Nutr Exerc Metab 2010;20(2): 132–8.
118. Anitua E, Andía I, Sanchez M, et al. Autologous preparations rich in growth factors promote proliferation and induce VEGF and HGF production by human tendon cells in culture. J Orthop Res 2005;23(2):281–6.
119. Guha N, Dashwood A, Thomas NJ, et al. IGF-I abuse in sport. Curr Drug Abuse Rev 2009;2(3):263–72.
120. Creaney L, Hamilton B. Growth factor delivery methods in the management of sports injuries: the state of play. Br J Sports Med 2008;42(5):314–20.
121. Banfi G, Corsi MM, Volpi P. Could platelet rich plasma have effects on systemic circulating growth factors and cytokine release in orthopaedic applications? Br J Sports Med 2006;40(10):816.

Eating for Performance: Bringing Science to the Training Table

Leslie J. Bonci, MPH, RD, CSSN, LDN

KEYWORDS

• Nutrition • Sports medicine • Training • Athletes

Nutrition for athletes is a critical part of health and performance. Despite many advances in nutritional knowledge and dietary practices, sports nutrition-associated issues, such as fatigue, loss of strength and stamina, loss of speed, and problems with weight management and inadequate energy intake, continue to be common. Athletes want to optimize their athletic performance and are willing to work tirelessly to achieve it. Yet, sound nutritional practices and well-designed patterns of eating are not awarded the same priority as training and many athletes fail to recognize that poor eating habits or suboptimal hydration choices may detract from athletic performance. Those who care for athletes and active individuals must take an active role in their nutritional well-being. The goal is to help athletes to SHOP: Safeguard Health and Optimize Performance. This article reviews the present generally accepted principles for nutritional management in sport.

The importance of the sports nutrition message cannot be overstated. Ideally, all of the athlete's support system (family, coaches, sports medicine staff) need to reinforce and remind athletes about fuel and fluid timing, quantity, and choices throughout the season. Getting athletes to embrace this concept may require substantial work on the athlete's part with constant reminders from their care providers. As a starting point, athletes should be encouraged to log food and fluid intake faithfully so they can see what, when, and how much they eat and drink. Before talking to the athlete about fueling around the time of exercise, it is advisable to ask about the overall meal distribution during the day. Some athletes upload (the bulk of their calories consumed in the evening), some middle load (more calories consumed mid-day), and few early load (consuming the majority of calories early in the day). The problem with those who upload is that their physical activity occurs early in the day in the absence of adequate fuel, increasing the likelihood of fatigue and decreased performance parameters during exercise. Getting athletes to buy into the concept of eating earlier in the day

Sports Medicine Nutrition, Department of Orthopedic Surgery and the Center for Sports Medicine, University of Pittsburgh Medical Center, Center for Sports Medicine, 3200 South Water Street, Pittsburgh, PA 15203, USA
E-mail address: boncilj@upmc.edu

Clin Sports Med 30 (2011) 661–670
doi:10.1016/j.csm.2011.03.011
0278-5919/11/$ – see front matter © 2011 Elsevier Inc. All rights reserved.

sportsmed.theclinics.com

may be aided by emphasizing its positive impact on performance. Strength, speed, and stamina are clearly enhanced with adequate fuel rather than without. For athletes with early morning practice, eating before exercise may be problematic because of a lack of appetite or reluctance to have food in the stomach pre-exercise. It may be wise to recommend breakfast before bed as a way of ensuring that the athlete is prefueled before morning activity.

The most important component of eating for performance is the timing of food and fluid consumption relative to the time of exercise. Ideally, fueling and hydration occur before a body is physically active and not just in a competitive situation. When evaluating an athlete's nutritional practices, key questions include

What do you eat and drink before practice/competition?
When do you eat/drink before practice/competition?
What do you eat and drink during practice/competition?
What do you eat/drink after practice/competition?
How soon do you eat/drink after practice/competition?

Many athletes are guilty of improper preparation before sport in a variety of ways. Common deleterious practices that must be identified and corrected include consuming no or little food/fluid before exercise, relying on water alone for lengthy practices/conditioning sessions, waiting too long to refuel/rehydrate postexercise, picking the wrong dietary items, and avoiding certain foods/fluids that may be advantageous for fueling/recovery because of a mistaken belief that these items are bad.

PRE-EXERCISE

When talking to athletes about the timing of food/fluid before exercise, emphasis should be placed on the value of nutritional preparation as part of their warm-up, or prefuel. It is highly useful to approach the athlete with the idea of a fuel prescription to encourage them to prioritize eating and hydration around the time of exercise. It is also advisable to translate nutrients to food and numbers that give the athlete a readily appreciable frame of reference. For instance, many athletes do not know what 20 oz of fluid is, but they can readily relate to the volume of a standard water bottle. It is difficult for athletes to conceptualize 50 g of carbohydrate and 10 g of protein, but an 8-oz container of yogurt is a readily available energy source that contains both nutrients in the desired quantities.

For prefueling, the closer the time to activity the smaller the amount of food recommended. In addition, foods that are more rapidly digested, such as gels, applesauce, gelatin, and sports drinks, are easier to consume and feel lighter in the gut than energy bars or a sandwich. Although fiber, fat, and protein are essential nutrients, consuming too much of them before exercise can result in gut discomfort and delayed gastric emptying. Examples of desirable dietary choices relative to the timing of exercise are included in **Table 1**.

Inquire as to what athletes can tolerate and what dietary preferences they have. Some may say they are too tired or nervous to chew. It is vital that these athletes learn to make choices that will allow them to work around their uneasiness about eating or drinking. A concentrated sports drink or a small smoothie, for example, can fuel without weighing them down or generating discomfort during sport.

DURING EXERCISE

During exercise, the purpose of caloric intake is obviously to remain fueled for sustained high-level physical activity. However, many athletes consume nothing but water

Table 1 Food choices for exercise	
Time of Exercise (h)	**Food Choices**
3–4	Turkey sandwich Pasta Waffles/eggs Stir fry of rice, vegetables, and chicken
2	Fruit and yogurt Bowl of cereal
<1	Gelatin Small smoothie Half bagel with honey or jam
Back-to-back events	Sports drink Half of bagel with jam or honey Half of a sports bar Applesauce Oatmeal with brown sugar or maple syrup

during daily practice/conditioning sessions. This practice can be problematic because athletes often work harder in training than they do in competition, yet they consume no calories during training. Ideally, carbohydrate feeding should occur shortly after the start of exercise. A sports drink is ideal because it provides fuel in addition to fluid and electrolytes. The current recommendation is for 30 to 60 g of carbohydrate per hour of endurance exercise.[1,2] For activity less than 1 hour in duration, water or a sports drink will generally suffice.[3–5] Not every athlete requires a sports beverage, but the following individuals may benefit from using them:

- Those who do not or cannot consume a pre-exercise meal
- Those who skip a meal or meals throughout the day
- Those who participate in intense training of several hours duration
- Those who participate in 2 or more training sessions per day.

RECOVERY NUTRITION

After exercise, the nutritional goal is to refuel to replace muscle glycogen and prepare for the next practice or competition, which is commonly referred to as recovery nutrition. Recovery intake is not intended to be a meal but rather an appetizer or snack to help the repletion process occur sooner rather than later. In general, the recommendation is to start to refuel within 30 to 60 minutes of exercise cessation to encourage higher glycogen levels postexercise.[6] Some have referred to this as the golden hour of energy repletion. Depending on exercise intensity or duration, however, recovery nutrition is not always necessary. A swimmer who is tapering or a lightweight workout would not warrant aggressive recovery nutrition because of a low level of energy consumption. Short workouts, light workouts, having adequate time for recovery, and during times of training taper are all circumstances where recovery nutrition may not be warranted.

Putting this all together, eating for performance occurs along a continuum. Ideally athletes fuel throughout the day and are continuously supplementing their caloric intake based on the timing and intensity of their training or competition. Note in **Table 2** the unique distribution of calorie consumption for an athlete as compared with the general population.

Table 2
Food choices for rest and activity

Basic eating:	Breakfast	Lunch	Dinner
Sports eating:	Breakfast	Lunch	Dinner
+Add ins:	Pre-exercise/ postexercise	Pre-exercise/ postexercise	Snack if needed OR Breakfast before bed for early AM workouts

The general recommendation is 0.5 g of carbohydrate per pound body weight (BW) after the workout. For a 150-lb athlete, they would need to consume 75 g of carbohydrate, which may be provided by

- A bagel and 20 oz of sports drink OR
- A bar, such as Zone, Power, or Clif, with a piece of fruit and water OR
- 12 oz of low-fat chocolate milk and a small handful of pretzels.

This recovery nutrition gives the athlete time to cool down, relax, and regain an appetite so that the subsequent meal can be eaten and enjoyed, not rapidly consumed en route to the next event of the day. Those who will benefit most from recovery nutrition include athletes who are involved in tournaments or multiple competitions over the course of several days, athletes who participate in multiple workouts per day, athletes who skip meals, athletes who do not consume adequate calories at baseline, athletes who need to gain strength and power, and athletes who need to improve endurance capacity.

There is often a question about the need or rationale for consuming protein along with carbohydrates postexercise. In athletes who have trouble meeting their daily protein requirements, consuming protein postexercise certainly helps them reach their daily goal. Research suggests that consuming 20 g of protein 5 to 6 times per day may be preferable to larger protein intake less frequently.[7]

Appropriate recovery foods with a favorable mix of carbohydrate and protein include

- Yogurt with granola
- Crackers, cheese, and fruit
- A small smoothie
- 2 small handfuls of trail mix
- A bagel with soy nut, almond, or peanut butter and jam or honey.

CALORIE REQUIREMENTS

Every athlete needs to operate within an appropriate calorie range to maximize performance, aid in physical development, control weight, and maintain health. However, some athletes routinely underconsume or overconsume calories, and few get it right consistently. This practice may lead to fatigue and decreased performance as well as adverse changes in body composition. Effective advice for athletes on setting calorie goals is to reinforce that their needs are greater than sedentary people, however, their needs are not limitless. Using a prediction equation can individualize calorie requirements with allowance for fluctuations in intensity of activity. The Harris-Benedict equation is the one most often used to determine basic calorie requirements.[8,9]

Men: $662 - 9.53 \times A + PA [15.91(W + 539.6H)]$

Women: $354 - 6.91 \times A + PA [9.36(W) + 726(H)]$

A = age
W = weight in kilograms
H = height in centimeters
PA = Physical activity
    1.0 to 1.39: Sedentary/light
    1.4 to 1.59: Daily living activity + 30 to 60 minutes of exercise per day
    1.6 to 1.89: Active (60 minutes of exercise daily)
    1.9 to 2.5: Very active (<60 minutes of moderate + 60 minutes of vigorous exercise daily OR <120 minutes of moderate daily activity).

Although the Harris-Benedict formula may be an effective way of determining calorie requirements for those performing moderate exercise, it will underestimate calorie requirements for athletes engaged in more than 1 hour of activity daily. The following estimates may be more appropriate for such an athletic population:

• Female athletes: 17 to 20 cal/lb BW
• Male athletes: 19 to 23 cal/lb BW
• Those recovering from injury: 15 cal/lb BW
• Those in low-intensity activities or exercising 3 to 5 days per week: 17 to 19 cal/lb BW
• Those who train several hours per day, 5 days per week + conditioning 2 to 3 days per week: 18 to 20 cal/lb BW
• Rigorous daily training: 19 to 23 cal/lb BW
• Triathlon training/nonelite: 22 to 25 cal/lb BW
• Competitive marathoners and triathletes: 25 to 30 cal/lb BW.

Even when athletes know their relative calorie range, they still need guidance on how to consume the appropriate types and quantities of calories each day for sport. One of the best online tools is the US Department of Agriculture Web site: www.mypyramidtracker.gov. This Web site can be an excellent educational tool for athletes with inadequate calorie consumption and also serves as a useful visual reminder to those who are overconsuming calories.

HYDRATION

Athletes know they need to be well hydrated, but confusion abounds. What is a fluid? How much is the right amount? What if an athlete is not thirsty? On average, daily fluid losses are greater than 2 L/d and an athlete who trains 2 hours a day can lose an additional 2 to 3 L of fluid. Athletes with large sweat losses may find it extremely difficult to take in enough fluid during exercise to maintain a reasonable fluid balance. This point is especially important in warm weather, where fluid requirements may reach 10+ L/d.[10] The National Academies of Science, Institute of Medicine released fluid guidelines in 2007,[11] which include

• Women: 91 oz/d: food + fluid
    72 oz through fluid (eg, nine 8-oz glasses of fluid)
• Men: 125 oz/d: food + fluid
    100 oz of fluid (eg, twelve 8-oz glasses of fluid).

These guidelines are for basic fluid needs but do not incorporate fluid guidelines for physical activity. The American College of Sports Medicine Position Stand on Fluid Replacement during Exercise 2004[12] addresses fluid guidelines pre-exercise, during, and postexercise. Athletes need to realize that fluid requirements will vary depending upon sweat rate, season, level of intensity, frequency, and duration of exercise. In addition, gastrointestinal (GI) tolerance of fluid during exercise is a major factor. The athlete who feels that their stomach is overly full is not going to be comfortable consuming fluids while active. Consequently, it is vital to have athletes train their guts to adapt to drinking while physically active. This practice is a key part of preparation for athletic success. All of the following constitute viable fluid choices for athletes: water, fitness waters, sports drinks, juice, milk, coffee, tea, carbonated beverages, energy drinks, and soups.

Athletes need to think about hydration before they are active. If possible, 4 hours pre-exercise they should consume 2 to 3 mL/lb body weight.[12] For a 150-lb athlete, this equates to 300 to 450 mL or approximately 12 to 16 oz (1.5–2.0 c) of fluid. If the athlete does not urinate within 2 hours of this fluid consumption, an additional 2 to 3 mL/lb BW is recommended.[12] Gastric emptying is maximized when the amount of fluid in the stomach is higher pre-exercise. Consuming fluids before exercise initiates both physiologic and hormonal responses that function to maintain the sweat rate by stimulating heat loss during exercise.[13,14] It is difficult for athletes to match their sweat loss with fluid intake during exercise because gastric emptying during exercise is slowed and unlikely to exceed 2 L/h. Thus, the goal of drinking fluid during exercise is not to achieve complete repletion of losses but rather to prevent excessive dehydration and excessive changes in electrolyte balance.[12] This is also why some individuals may need to consume sports drinks (as opposed to water only) during exercise, especially those who are salty sweaters. As such, calculating one's individual sweat rate may be beneficial:

Weight (pre-exercise) − Weight (postexercise) in ounces (16 oz = 1 lb)
+
Number of ounces of fluid consumed during exercise
÷
Number of hours of exercise =
Hourly sweat rate or number of ounces of fluid athlete should drink per hour of exercise

Example

150-lb soccer player loses 32 oz (2 lb) during practice, exercises for 2 hours, drinks 20 oz of fluid during practice
150 − 148 = 2 lb or 32 oz (2 × 16)
+
20 oz fluid intake
÷
2 = 26 oz of fluid required per hour

Knowing their sweat rate number allows athletes to plan accordingly with regards to consuming enough liquid per hour. In light of the previous numbers, more than 1 bottle of fluid is probably necessary for most athletes. Calculating the sweat rate is simple, cheap, and should be done periodically throughout the season especially with changes in weather. Helpful tips to optimize fluid intake include

- Bring fluid. You cannot drink what you do not have.
- Drink early and often, from the moment they wake up.
- Start practice with a comfortably full stomach.
- Remind athletes that 1 gulp from a water fountain is approximately 1 oz.
- Practice hydration during training.
- Hydrate with fluid in, not ON the body.
- Drink fluid with meals.
- Drink during exercise; larger gulps may be better tolerated than sips and result in less gastric fullness.

After exercise, there are several strategies that can be used for rehydration. Rapid rehydration with water alone occurs over 12 to 24 hours.[10,15–17] However, the athlete who consumes water alone may not drink enough because water may blunt the thirst mechanism and result in cessation of fluid consumption before needs are met. The general guidelines are to consume 20 oz of fluid (fluid or fluid + food) for every pound lost during exercise. When more rapid rehydration is warranted, a sports beverage is preferred because it provides fluid, carbohydrates, and electrolytes. An alternative is to consume water and a food that contains carbohydrates and electrolytes, such as pretzels.[18]

IRON

Iron depletion is more prevalent in female athletes,[19] and iron requirements for endurance athletes may be increased by at least 70% relative to nonendurance athletes.[20,21] Athletes experience higher rates of iron deficiency than nonathletes as a result of iron losses in the sweat, iron losses in the GI tract, foot strike hemolysis in runners, and losses associated with menstruation. Additional nutritional contributors to depleted iron include

- Decreased energy/protein intake
- Poor absorptive capacity
- Fad diets
- Heavy sweat loss
- Food insecurity (access/availability)
- Use of laxatives
- Fasting
- Excessive consumption of tea, coffee, and other iron-binding foods/fluids.

The major concern for athletes is that iron deficiency or iron deficiency anemia is performance impairing. They can result in a variety of deleterious symptoms, including fatigue exacerbated by exertion, dyspnea, increased lethargy/sleepiness/apathy, poor concentration, moodiness/irritability, increased susceptibility to injury, and complaints of feeling cold. Athletes at highest risk include female athletes, dieters and those who restrict calories, vegetarian athletes, athletes who are involved in a more intense training regimen than usual, and athletes who are frequent blood donors.

The solution to iron deficiency is not just iron supplementation but also an assessment of intake and recommendations for iron-containing foods. The dietary reference intake for iron is 15 to 18 mg/d, but the recommendation for athletes is at least 18 mg/d for both men and women. Vegetarian athletes may require up to 1.8 times the daily requirement for iron.[21] Athletes may increase iron intake through a variety of dietary sources:

- Iron-fortified cereals, such as TOTAL, consumed with a vitamin C source to facilitate absorption
- Iron-fortified breads
- Meat, especially red meat and dark meat of poultry
- Spinach with strawberries to increase absorption
- Chili made with beef or dark meat of turkey, beans, and tomatoes
- Noodles with a marinara sauce
- Nuts and dried fruit.

If the athlete is trying to increase iron-containing foods or needs to take iron supplements, they should follow the provided guidelines to ensure that they are maximizing absorption of iron from their diet:

- Space out polyphenols (tannins) from tea, coffee, red wine, or cocoa from iron supplements
- Space out phytate consumption with iron supplements: whole grains, wheat bran, wheat germ, seeds, soy foods, oatmeal, and lentils
- Space out iron supplements from high-fiber cereals
- Separate timing of iron and calcium supplements because calcium may affect iron absorption
- Separate timing of zinc or magnesium supplements from iron
- Limit consumption of high-oxalate foods with iron supplements: spinach, rhubarb, Swiss chard, dark chocolate, and beer.

Athletes should be tested not only for hemoglobin levels but also serum ferritin, a more sensitive measure of iron status. If the values are low, a starting point is to supplement with an iron-containing multivitamin plus iron-containing food with a goal of adding at least 20 additional milligrams per day. If an iron supplement is necessary, ferrous sulfate is advised, starting with 1 tablet that provides 35 to 60 mg of elemental iron. If iron deficiency anemia is present, 2 tablets are recommended: 1 in the morning, 1 in the evening. The ultimate goal is to replete iron via foods (noted later) not just iron supplementation. An increase in the dietary intake has been shown to be more effective than 50 mg of iron supplementation in protecting hemoglobin and serum ferritin in young women.[22] Common sources of iron are included in **Table 3**.

The United States Olympic Committee has an iron deficiency prevention protocol that addresses iron supplementation for athletes training at sea level and at altitude.[23]

Table 3
Iron content of foods

Food	Portion	Fe (mg)
Hamburger	3 oz patty	3
Roast beef	3 oz	3
Steak	6 oz	9
Turkey/chicken	3 oz	3
Dark meat	—	—
Tuna	3 oz	2
Ham	3 oz	2
Pizza[a]	1 slice	3
Beans/lentils[a]	1 c cooked	2
Eggs	2	2
Bagel[a]	1	2
Cereal with iron[a]	1 c	3
Waffle/pancake[a]	1	3
Raisins[a]	¼ c	2.5
Spinach[a]	1 c raw	3
Nuts or seeds[a]	¼ c	1

[a] Plant-based (nonheme) iron sources are absorbed better in conjunction with vitamin C-containing foods/beverages.

Even with supplementation, improving the diet is the first step in learning to resolve iron deficiency. It is important to remind athletes to add iron slowly to minimize GI distress and to consume plant-based sources of iron with vitamin C-containing foods/beverages to increase absorption.

SUMMARY

Keeping athletes safe and optimizing performance are hallmarks of sports medicine practice. Reinforcing the message of adequate nutrition as part of this philosophy should be accomplished at the time of the preparticipation physical examination, during routine visits, and with other interactions with athletes. Asking "how are you eating?" may be enough of a prompt to reprioritize the importance of sound nutrition for athletes. Appropriate nutrition provides the edge for improved strength, speed, stamina, and recovery. Proper caloric intake ensures that athletes are optimally fueled for their sport and, for younger athletes, optimizes proper growth and development. The importance of hydration cannot be overemphasized and needs to be part of every encounter with athletes. Assessing iron status and educating about iron intake can help athletes to improve on the field as well as in the workplace or classroom.

As care providers for athletes, it is essential that we understand the basic principles of food and fluid use in athletes and that we can identify deficiencies. Use of sound scientific principles should maximize an athlete's nutritional status and enhance performance and health.

REFERENCES

1. Coggan AR, Coyle EF. Carbohydrate ingestion during prolonged exercise: effects on metabolism and performance. Exerc Sport Sci Rev 1991;19:1–20.
2. Currell K, Jeukendrup AE. Superior endurance performance with ingestion of multiple transportable carbohydrates. Med Sci Sports Exerc 2008;40:275–81.
3. Suguira K, Kobayashi K. effect o carbohydrate ingestion on sprint performance following continuous and intermittent exercise. Med Sci Sports Exerc 1998;30:1624–30.
4. Jeukendrup A, Brouns F, Wagenmakers AJ, et al. Carbohydrate-electrolyte feedings improve 1 h time trial cycling performance. Int J Sports Med 1997;18:125–9.
5. Nicholas CW, Williams C, Lakony HK, et al. Influence of ingesting a carbohydrate–electrolyte solution on endurance capacity during intermittent, high-intensity shuttle running. J Sports Sci 1995;13:283–90.
6. Ivy JL, Katz AL, Cutler CL, et al. Muscle glycogen synthesis after exercise. Effect of time of carbohydrate ingestion. J Appl Physiol 1988;64:1480–5.
7. Moore DR, Robinson MJ, Fry JL, et al. Ingested protein dose response of muscle and albumin protein synthesis after resistance exercise in young men. Am J Clin Nutr 2009;89:161–8.
8. Frankenfield DC, Rowe WA, Smith JS, et al. Validation of several established equations for resting metabolic rate in obese and non obes people. J Am Diet Assoc 2003;103:1152–9.
9. Institute of Medicine. Dietary Reference intakes for energu, carbohydrate, fiber, fat, protein and amino acids (macronutrients). Washington, DC: National Academy Press; 2002. Available at: http://www.nap.edu. Accessed March 16, 2011.
10. Maughan RJ, Shirreffs SM, Galloway DR, et al. Dehydration and fluid replacement in sport and exercise. Sports Exerc Inj 1995;1:148–53.

11. Institute of Medicine. Dietary reference intakes for waterm potassium, sodium and chloride. Washington, DC: National Academy Press; 2004. Available at: http://www.nap.edu. Accessed March 16, 2011.
12. American College of Sports Medicine. Exercise and fluid replacement. Med Sci Sports Exerc 2007;39:377–90.
13. Montain SJ, Coyle EF. The influence of graded dehydration on hyperthermia and cardiovascular drift durin exercise. J Appl Physiol 1992;73:1340–50.
14. Verbalis JG. Inhibitory controls of drinking: satiation of thirst. In: Ramsay DJ, Booth DA, editors. Thirst: physiological and psychological aspects. London: Springer-Verlag; 1991. p. 315–7.
15. Maughan R, Leiper JB, Shirreffs SM. Rehydration and recovery after exercise. Sports Sci Exch 1996;9:1–4. Available at: http://www.gssiweb.org. Accessed March 16, 2011.
16. Nadel ER, Mack GW, Nose H. Influence of fluid replacement beverages on body fluid homeostasis during exercise and recovery. In: Gisolfi CV, Lamb DR, editors. Perspectives in exercise science and sports medicine; fluid homeostasis during exercise. Indianapolis (IN): Benchmark Press; 1988. p. 195.
17. Nadel ER. New ideas for rehydration beverages during and after exercise in hot weather. Sports Sci Exch 1988;1:1–5.
18. Schedl HP, Maughan RJ, Gisolfi CV. Intestinal absorption during rest and exercise: implications for formulating an oral rehydration solution. Med Sci Sports Exerc 1994;26:267–80.
19. Beard J, Tobin B. Iron status and exercise. AJCN 2000;72(2):594S–7S.
20. Whiting SJ, Barabash WA. Dietary Reference Intakes for the micronutrients. Considerations for physical activity. Appl Physiol Nutr Metab 2006;31:80–5.
21. Institute of Medicine. Food and nutrition board. Dietary reference intakes for vitamin a, vitamin k, arsenic, boron, chromium, copper, iodine, iron, manganese, molybdenum, nickel, silicon, vanadium and zinc. Washington, DC: National Academies Press; 2001.
22. Lyle RM, Weaver CM, Sedlock DA, et al. Iron status in exercising women: the effectof oral iron therapy vs increased consumption of muscle foods. Am J Clin Nutr 1992;56:1049–55.
23. United States Olympic Committee Iron Deficiency Protocol. Available at: http://www.teamusa.org/iron_deficiency_prevention_protocol. Accessed March 16, 2011.

FURTHER READINGS

Bonci LJ. Sport nutrition for coaches. Champaign (IL): Human Kinetics; 2009.
Dunford M, editor. Sports nutrition: a practice manual for professionals. 4th edition. Chicago (IL): SCAN Dietetic Practice Group, American Dietetic Association; 2006.
Rodriguez NR, DiMarco NM, Langley S. Position of the American dietetic association, dietitians of Canada and the American College of Sports Medicine: nutrition and athletic performance. J Am Diet Assoc 2009;109(3):509–27.

Index

Note: Page numbers of article titles are in **boldface** type.

A

Acne, treatment of, 633–634
Alcohol, use by athletes, 620, 652
Allergic rhinitis, treatment of, 632
Anemia, iron deficiency, 667
Anti-doping policies, updates on, 650–653
Antibiotics, for athletes, 632–633
   oral, in acne, 634
   topical, in acne, 633
Antidepressants, increased use of, 634
Antimicrobial agents, in acne, 633
Anxiety disorders, and normal anxiety, distinguished, 617
   in athletes, 616–618
Aorta, descending thoracic, dissection of, 508
Aortic valve, bicuspid, familial, 518
Arterial vasodilation, endothelium-dependent, 552
Asthma, medications in, 631–632
Athlete(s), elite, cardiovascular screening in, **503–524**
      concepts and controversy in, 505–507
      diagnostic testing and, 509
      electrocardiography in, 509–512, 513, 515, 516, 519
      history and physical examination initiating, 507–508
      view of future in, 516–521
   with special needs, preparticipation physical examination for, 499
Athlete's pharmacy, **629–639**
Attention-deficit hyperactivity disorder, and athlete, **591–610**
   as heterogenous behavioral disorder, 592
   athletes with, 598
   causes of, 595–597
   childhood onset of, 593, 618
   definition of, 592
   diagnosis of, 594
      in college years, 597–598
   effect of sport on, 599
   effect on sport, 598–599
   functional impairment in, 595, 635
   impairment in, 593
   in college athlete, 591, 618
   inattention and/or overactivity/impulsivity (hyperactivity) in, 592–593
   incidence of, 597
   medications used to treat, 599–601
      cardiac safety and, 605

Clin Sports Med 30 (2011) 671–678
doi:10.1016/S0278-5919(11)00047-0
0278-5919/11/$ – see front matter © 2011 Elsevier Inc. All rights reserved.

sportsmed.theclinics.com

Moving?

Make sure your subscription moves with you!

To notify us of your new address, find your **Clinics Account Number** (located on your mailing label above your name), and contact customer service at:

Email: journalscustomerservice-usa@elsevier.com

800-654-2452 (subscribers in the U.S. & Canada)
314-447-8871 (subscribers outside of the U.S. & Canada)

Fax number: 314-447-8029

Elsevier Health Sciences Division
Subscription Customer Service
3251 Riverport Lane
Maryland Heights, MO 63043

*To ensure uninterrupted delivery of your subscription, please notify us at least 4 weeks in advance of move.

Printed and bound by CPI Group (UK) Ltd, Croydon, CR0 4YY

03/10/2024

01040454-0017